MW00513168

The Seasons of Good-bye: An Alzheimer's Caregiver Journal

Robyn Feld

Halian Associates
Maplewood, MN

The Seasons of Good-bye: An Alzheimer's Caregiver Journal copyright © 2005 by Robyn Feld.
All rights reserved. Printed in Eagan, MN, U.S.A. No part of this book may be used or reproduced in
any manner whatsoever without written permission except in the case of reprints in the context of reviews.
For information, write Halian Associates, 1292 Ferndale St. N.
Maplewood, MN 55119

All anecdotes contained in this book were freely shared by Alzheimer's caregivers. Because each AD patient has
individual needs, any care process or procedure outlined in this book should be discussed with medical personnel or
professional caregivers before implementing.

ISBN: 0-9759762-0-6

Library of Congress Control Number: 2004095389

Book design by Robyn Feld

Dedication

This book is dedicated, with admiration and respect, to AD caregivers everywhere. A very special "thank you" to those who so freely shared their experiences with me so that, together, we can help other caregivers:

Jackie N.	Marian L.
RW	Marie T.
Carl E.	Neita D.
Joyce J.	Marion A.
Gerry T.	Peggy H.
Margaret B.	Mary A.
Laura F.	Dee C.
Lee C.	Del R.
Carol H.	Lois K.
Mary Ann S.	Mary K.
Beth W.	Gail S.
Lynn R.	Sharon M.
Nonya C.	

Their candid reflections on the Alzheimer's caregiver journey are the heart of this book. I have not edited their responses except to enhance readability as needed.

Acknowledgements

I lost my Mom to AD on December 16, 2002. She suffered for many years and, as her only child, I was her main caregiver. I wrote this book to be the resource I wished I had had at that time.

When I got the idea to put this book together, I knew I would be running the project on sheer heart as opposed to publishing know-how. Every aspect of the production was a learning experience! I cannot thank my support team enough:

~ My wonderful children, Scott Feld and Wendy Neer, and their families. They watched their Nana fade away because of AD and their support for this project was heartening.

~ My aunt, Jackie Nelson, who walked her sister's AD journey with me and has become one of my dearest friends.

~ My good friend, Marian Lensegrav, who pioneered the AD journey for me as her mother's caregiver. She shared both her pain during her mother's illness and the knowledge gained afterward in order to help me with my Mom.

~ Other friends and family who cheered me on - everyone at CPPNA, the Feld clan (especially Margaret), Irene Jansen, the Crawfords, Judi Schellenberg, Jane Schoen, Kim Johnson, Vickie Husa, my Melaleuca friends and others, who, with a kind word or encouraging e-mail, kept my spirits up.

I am pleased to donate $1.00 from the sale of each book to Alzheimer's outreach and research.

Robyn Feld

This book belongs to _____

to help with care for _____

Short Table of Contents

SPRING – Remembering The Person Before AD

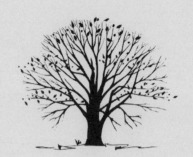

Appearance

_____

_____

_____

_____

_____

_____

_____

_____

_____

_____

_____

_____

_____

_____

_____

_____

Immediate family (parents, siblings, others)

_____

_____

_____

_____

_____

_____

_____

_____

_____

_____

_____

_____

_____

_____

Married with children (or not)

_____
_____
_____
_____
_____
_____
_____
_____
_____
_____
_____
_____
_____
_____
_____
_____

Faith-based activities

_____

_____

_____

_____

_____

_____

_____

_____

_____

_____

_____

_____

_____

_____

_____

Having fun

Celebrations and holidays

Doing for others (volunteerism, caregiving, etc.)

Quirks, mannerisms, hobbies, etc.

Friends and neighbors

Education

Childhood

Favorite foods to prepare and/or eat

_____

_____

_____

_____

_____

_____

_____

_____

_____

_____

_____

_____

_____

_____

Memorable travels

Other Memories

_____

_____

_____

_____

_____

_____

_____

_____

_____

_____

_____

_____

_____

_____

_____

SUMMER – The Diagnosis

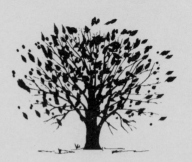

How the diagnosis was made

~ I lived with Mom from 1971 to 1991 when she died. I notice strange symptoms in the early 80's. I took her to a neurologist who asked her to repeat words at short intervals. He felt I should wait a few weeks and write down observations at home. When I went back, I believe he took a brain scan – ruled out other diseases and was sure it was the beginning stages. Mom was 79 at the time.

Marie's daughter, MN

~ Mom was living in Tucson, AZ and I was not there when she was diagnosed at the U of A shortly after my Dad died in 1988. She was just forgetful. She was medicated with a medicine that she was taken off of because it affected her liver. She was 88 when diagnosed.

Milta's son, KS

~ My mother dearly loved shopping and was glad when we took her. When she suddenly demanded everything be returned to the store, we were shocked. At a visit to the doctor, I told him this and was informed by him that this was dementia and would lead into Alzheimer's.

Mary's daughter, MN

~ Gerald knew his memory was worsening. Our family doctor started him on antidepressant and artery-opening medications. He had a CAT scan in 1994. In the fall of 1996, I took him to a memory assessment clinic and to a neuropsychologist. Diagnosis: Alzheimer's, probably to a nursing home within a year. Was on Cognex [early AD drug].

Gerald's wife, IA

~ My Dad had a stroke and an EEG brain scan showed not only the stroke but that he had Alzheimer's. Like some others, we overlooked signs of the disease, probably not wanting to deal with the fact that our parents are aging and that they have health issues that need attention and in-home care.

Roy's daughter, MN

~ My sister and I liked to play cards. One day, she picked up her cards and said, "I've never played this before." We had been playing the same game on a regular basis for years. Another symptom showed up when we would go out to eat. She just sat there with the menu in front of her and wouldn't pick it up until I reminded her.

Lanie's sister, MN

~ My doctor would ask him questions she knew he knew but couldn't answer. She put him on Aricept, which did help some. In March, 2003, he didn't know where he was and couldn't find the bathroom, etc.

Clarence's wife, SC

~ Mom's primary-care doctor evaluated her for memory loss and referred her to a "geriatrician". I was with her when she was tested – it was very sad. He told her she had AD and would need assistance to live in five years. The doctor prescribed Reminal but Mom became depressed and anorexic so it had to be discontinued.   Ann's daughter, MN

~ My wife, Reatha, was diagnosed in 1990 at the age of 55 which puts her in the early-onset stage of Alzheimer's. Early-onset is supposed to progress faster than late-onset but it seems to be taking its own sweet time. We had been married for 36 years at that time and I really hadn't noticed any changes in my wife, as so often happens. Our son came home from college one weekend and was trying to play cards with his mother. He asked me what was wrong and I said I had no idea. Reatha had been a very good bridge player for many years. I had recently lost a good job because I was ignorant of the computer and had just taken a job with Dr. L., a psychiatrist, filing insurance claims. There was also a psychologist in the same office and when I talked to them about my wife, they both wanted to get her right in. They gave her all the tests, took X-ray tests hoping to find something treatable. No such luck – both finally agreed it was probably early-onset Alzheimer's disease. Neither one of us really understood what we were facing. Reatha's husband, IA

~ In 1999, I started going with my Mom to all of her doctor appointments. At her yearly physical, her doctor alerted me about the possibility of dementia. After some simple tests, he directed me to get information about Alzheimer's. By her next exam, 6 months later, Aricept was prescribed. At this time, it was suggested to look into some form of assisted living.   Myra's daughter, MN

~ We noticed changes in my mother's memory and some poor judgment and decision-making changes. We took her to a neurologist who believed it was early stages of Alzheimer's. My father died several years earlier and we had hoped she was displaying signs of grieving.   Mary's stepdaughter, MN

~ In the year preceding diagnosis, my Mom or my sisters would call me and mention "strange things" Grandma was doing or saying. She was always a meticulous housekeeper but was getting "messy" (a little). She also had unusual attacks of paranoia – she was afraid she had been sitting with my niece and nephews (she was not) and called my Mom in panic that she'd lost or misplaced them. A short while later, they became "kids" as I think she could no longer recall their names.   Gen's granddaughter, CA

~ Mom had always been eccentric so I believe she had the disease for years before being formally diagnosed with a verbal quiz by my doctor. We were too used to her quirky behavior to look for anything organic to be causing it, until it got out of hand. The doctor prescribed Aricept to try and slow Mom's decline. Also, Mom had an EEG (brain scan) to be sure that there was no other organic reason for her dementia.

Lanie's daughter, MN

YOUR THOUGHTS -

_____

_____

_____

_____

_____

_____

_____

_____

_____

_____

_____

_____

_____

Intellect is a man's guard; without it, he is like an infant. (proverb)

How the patient accepted the reality of AD

~ My mother was always more quiet and laid back. She never talked about it – in fact I think I was the only one the doctor spoke to using the term "Alzheimer's". He suggested readings – *The 36 Hour Day* [by Nancy L. Mace & Peter V. Rabins]. She knew she was forgetting more but did not seem unduly upset.
Marie's daughter, MN

~ Did he ever accept it?
Joe's wife, IA

~ He really did not verbalize things that were happening to him and was quick to deny that he did or said anything wrong. He would cover his confusion by remaining silent at times. He would occasionally become angry when things wouldn't go together for him. For instance, playing cards – it was always someone else's fault when the outcome wasn't right.
Joe's daughter, IA

~ My dad always would tell Mother that she had a good memory but it was awfully short. She would tell that about herself.
Margaret's daughter, KS

~ She knew she was failing mentally as her own mother had. She was aware she could no longer cook, sew, drive, handle money, etc. She said other people thought she was "crazy". She was very unhappy with herself.
Mildred's daughter, IA

~ In the nursing home one day, Mom asked us if she had Alzheimer's. This was the first and only time she mentioned it. Not sure if she realized what it was.
Mary's daughter, MN

~ Gerald was told he had Alzheimer's. He would look at some of the AD literature. When people asked him how he was, he'd say, "Great, but my memory is gone." Sometimes, he would say he was better now; that he didn't have AD anymore. He voluntarily gave up woodworking.
Gerald's wife, IA

~ Dad will not talk of the disease except he does acknowledge that his brain isn't working right and that it is caused from his "old age". He has admitted and discussed that his parents and grandparents had AD (only his Mom was diagnosed).
Roy's daughter, MN

~ Mom knew she was getting "forgetful" but never said anything beyond that.
Donna's daughter, IA

~ Mom only vaguely remembers the evaluation and seems unaware of the diagnosis. She is very aware of how difficult it is to remember things and think of words but she attributes it to the "shock" of the move from her house [to her apartment] "just agony". She will say in frustration,"What is wrong with my brain?"   Ann's daughter, MN

~ Mom knew her memory was failing and we would talk about it. It was like a fog coming over her mind. A very difficult time for her. But you stay close and work through each step as it comes. Being retired was a big plus for me.
Myra's daughter, MN

~ We were informed about Carol's disease by the mail sent to Carol. I was very angry about how the doctors chose to inform us. And, of course, it put Carol in a very deep state of depression for a while. Along with the antidepressant medication, Aricept and many conversations that we (the family) will be there for her, Carol has accepted her disease and is coping quite well. She jokes if someone forgets, that maybe they should take one of her Aricept pills.
Carol's husband, MN

~ My Mom hid symptoms from us – we had our own ideas that things were not right and tried to talk with her about money, pans left to burn on the stove, etc. When she couldn't identify family photos any longer, I was stunned. I knew at that point that part of my mother was lost to us – hidden somewhere I couldn't reach.   Genevieve's daughter, MN

~ My mother was not told of her diagnosis by either her children or her physician. She argued nothing was wrong, even when her dementia was severe.   Mary's stepdaughter, MN

~ Mom never accepted that she had Alzheimer's. "There's nothing wrong with me" and variations of that statement were what we heard over and over even though she now was too scared to drive and could not reliably prepare a meal for herself. But, being a very stubborn woman all her life and never wanting to rely on others, she insisted she was fine. After a few months, she did, from time to time, express something like "my head is not working right today" but this was temporarily in her mind, because at other times she would report that she was fine. When we tried to put a label on it, she would adamantly deny (usually with anger), saying "there's nothing wrong with me!" Helen's daughter, OR

~ My mother completely dismissed the findings and said the doctors were wrong. She became very upset and belligerent, adding it was not her, it was everyone else. It wasn't until the third year that she finally came to the realization of the disease.
Charlotte's daughter, TX

~ Mom was aware that she had Alzheimer's but did not discuss it except to say that *Readers Digest* had just had an article about it. This attitude did not surprise me as she had an aversion to talking about anything sad. The closest she ever came to talking about AD's effect on her was to say, "My brain isn't working right."

Lanie's daughter, MN

YOUR THOUGHTS –

_____

_____

_____

_____

_____

_____

_____

_____

_____

_____

_____

_____

_____

I'm just wandering. I think of things and then they go away.

(Iris Murdoch, AD victim; subject of film *Iris*, 2000)

How you, the caregiver, accepted the reality of AD

~ I was glad I did something about it but wasn't overly upset because I knew so little about it or how devastating it was. I think the big thing then was chicken soup – because they thought there was something in it that helped. The first stages dragged out so I went along with it.   Marie's daughter, MN

~ I accepted what it was and felt no guilt. We started going to meeting of support groups for caretakers – that really helped.   Alvin's wife, IA

~ I was aware of the disease but was not close to it until Mom came to live with us the last year of her life. She died in 1992 at our home.   Milta's son, KS

~ My Dad was her major caregiver. It was hurtful to see her so unhappy. It hurt the first time I visited and she didn't acknowledge me as someone special in her life.   Mildred's daughter, IA

~ I had more trouble accepting the diagnosis. I wanted her to be like she was before the disease and couldn't accept that she was slipping away from us.   Mary's daughter, MN

~ My sister and I were finally glad we had a diagnosis but my sister never admitted that Mom had the disease. We truly believe that other drugs could have been used, but we never questioned the doctors as to other drugs that could have been used.   Matilda's daughter, MN

~ I had to accept. I had to make all the decisions. I had to take care of him, the house, the car. I learned all I could about the disease – newspaper and magazine articles and books. I joined a support group (still go) and started another group. I attended any conferences or workshops I could find and talked with caregivers.   Gerald's wife, IA

~ Dad has been ill for years with other health issues and so the additional diagnosis of AD did not hit us so hard.   Roy's daughter, MN

~I have never been able to accept Alzheimer's. I believe in God and there are many terrible diseases in this world, but I don't understand why He would allow one that takes away one's mind and self-respect.   Lanie's sister, MN

~ I was finally told he was in the second stages of Alzheimer's. I took complete care of him from March until August.

Clarence's wife, SC

~ I was devastated by the diagnosis and had to find another living situation Mom would accept (she had put money down on a senior cooperative that had no meals or assisted living). The doctor said I had to make other arrangements. Mom was still in her own home when she was diagnosed.

Ann's daughter, MN

~ It was sad to watch such an interesting, loving person battle between two worlds and become so frustrated with herself.

Myra's daughter, MN

~ It's good to know what we are dealing with; that way, I can watch for changes as they occur. Fortunately, there are few right now – almost three years later.

Carol's husband, MN

~ I was somewhat comforted to realize my grandmother was not entirely aware of all that was happening to her/with her. It was almost a single moment in time when the reality of her diagnosis hit. My sister, Sue, called me and said, "Something is wrong with Grandma. Can you come right home?" I flew home within hours, spent the night with Grandma and knew instantly there was a serious problem. She was talking to long deceased relatives all night long. She had NO recognition of me.

Gen's granddaughter, CA

~ At first, I thought Mom's problem was depression due to Dad's death. After all, Mom had always kept to herself, had few friends and mostly had only us daughters as outside contact, generally speaking. After an unusually intimate conversation with her, Mom agreed she was depressed (a breakthrough!) and agreed to seek help. It was as if she knew there was a problem and was looking for someone to guide her toward the solution. This was one of the few times I saw Mom accepting the help/counsel of another. Once we had an AD diagnosis (due to the diligence of my sister's pursuits), I was relieved (we have a name) and scared for several reasons, including: 1.) There is no cure. 2.) Now what? 3.) It is hereditary – I'm at risk! 4.) I live 275 miles away – what am I supposed to do? (Thankfully, my sister was local.)

Helen's daughter, OR

~ It was very hard for me to accept the situation. She had allergic reactions (stomach-aches, hallucinations, etc.) to conventional medicine. Therefore, I pursued supplements and alternative medicine as prescribed by a naturopath. Mom improved for a while.

Helen's daughter, WA

~ I was glad to finally have a name for the behavior although it was the worst possible outcome. I was wracked with guilt for not getting her to a doctor sooner – it took me a long time to work through the "what-ifs". I was so grateful that the Aricept worked for Mom, at least for a little while: it doesn't work for everyone.   Lanie's daughter, MN

YOUR THOUGHTS -

It's rather like falling from stair to stair in series of bumps.

(John Bayley, author of *Iris*, about his wife's- Iris Murdoch - AD)

How everyday life was adjusted for the AD patient

~ The month of January was spent moving her out of her home of 35 years. It was horrendous! She is now in a senior apartment with the coin laundry down the hall, with meals available, plus other services that can be added. Half of the 4th floor is assisted living. My Mom has never lived in an apartment in her life. This is a huge adjustment. Ann's daughter, MN

~ Reatha was able to continue working another year or so until the number problem forced them to put her on disability. They took real good care of her until Social Security disability took over in two years. She was able to stay by herself for maybe the next year. Then she had a hard time telling reality from the TV she was watching. She was in the psych ward of our local hospital for a period of time. I realized now that she couldn't be left alone. Reatha had a very good friend that said she would be happy, and she was, to pick Reatha up at 8:00 a.m., take her to the mall and walk a while, then have coffee and a cookie. After that, she would take her to the Adult Day Care Center where she could stay 'til 3:00 p.m. when I had to arrange for someone to pick her up until I got off of work. After a period of time, our friends were getting harder to find to look after Reatha, and also the Day Center said they couldn't keep her much longer because she was becoming more agitated and needed one-on-one care. I hired a lady to stay with her until I could retire in 1995. Reatha's husband, IA

~ Every week, we set up a routine and wrote the schedule on the calendar. Very basic but helpful for Mom. We had a nurse and social worker come in to check Mom's home out for safety. We also set in place Mom's participating two days a week at Adult Day Services. It's a wonderful program. With still another organization, I lined up a lady to visit with Mom every Thursday afternoon. She would take Mom for a ride, read to her or just reminisce. Myra's daughter, MN

~ We had planned to do more traveling after we retired but Carol has difficulty dealing with strange surroundings. I now do make all financial decisions for us. She still enjoys shopping with her sisters on Saturdays. I make out the list and her sisters help her do this list. I do all of the grocery shopping and cooking now, although I did some of this before Carol was diagnosed. Carol's husband, MN

~ Mom was Dad's main caretaker. They had a friend that would take Dad out for the afternoon which would relieve Mom for a few hours. My sister and I did what we could to help. Alvin's daughter, IA

~ It came very quickly – a psychotic break, a day in the E.R., hospital admission for 3 days while my daughter and I made the rounds, searching for a long-term care facility. Mom never saw her lovely little apartment again. She never even asked about it – it was "erased" from her mind. Genevieve's daughter, MN

~ Mother lived in Superior [Wisconsin]. The closest children lived in St. Paul. I called the Dean at Superior State College and she found a foreign student who would live free at Mom's house. She did no caretaking but at least someone was in the house at night. Mother never really liked or accepted the student and was not nice to her. Later, we contacted a nursing agency and an aide came daily (9 a.m. to 8 p.m.) to be with Mom. At this point, she was not making meals, etc. My brother, sister and I came home very other weekend to shop, clean, etc. Mary's stepdaughter, MN

~ I don't know that we did anything different at home – he just remained in his chair most of the time. Joe's wife, IA

~ Some of us made excuses for his errors. Some corrected him but, for the most part, going along with him served the most useful method. He stopped driving on his own and towards the end of time at home, no longer went outside much. Mom pretty much waited on him. Joe's daughter, IA

~ My wife worked full time and I operated a business out of our home, so we arranged for adult day care at a local AD nursing home. It was 8-5 and it kept Mom busy during the day. During weekends and evenings, we would involve her in different activities. Milta's son, KS

~ Mother lived with us when she first came down from Minnesota (1994). Then into an apartment in a high rise and I would visit after work 2-3 times a week. She was in good spirits and was able to work as a foster grandparent at a daycare. Margaret's daughter, KS

~ For a time, Dad tried to cook and do everything. Both refused to have help. Things were really going to pot and they weren't eating right. House was overrun with cockroaches. Mom had no help with personal care or hygiene. They initially hired a housekeeper who was very caring and good. Mildred's daughter, IA

~ I would take Clarence grocery-store shopping but had to watch that he didn't wander off. He loved to go and talk to people in the store. I'm glad we were both retired and had traveled while we could and enjoyed it. Clarence's wife, SC

~ My aunt and I set up a regular schedule of taking Mom out for a meal and a car ride – she during the week and me on weekends. I also took Mom shopping on weekends. We tried to treat her as we always had but were constantly on guard for signs of decline. I did consider quitting work to live with Mom but I needed the income and benefits as I was supporting myself.

Lanie's daughter, MN

YOUR THOUGHTS -

_____

_____

_____

_____

_____

_____

_____

_____

_____

_____

_____

_____

How everyday life was adjusted for you, the caregiver

~ There were many phone calls after receiving a sweepstakes notification in the mail. Grandma was convinced she was the million-dollar winner. She whispered on the phone to keep the winning secret so others wouldn't try to "get some" (paranoia). I worried about her vulnerability to telemarketers and "con-men" (swindlers) – she was always so kind-hearted and willing to help. Since she lived in an apartment in a retirement community, I worried less about her personal safety than when she lived in her own home. Gen's granddaughter, CA

~ Because I was 275 miles away, my contact was not daily but my visits increased to about every six weeks. I also called most every day. Until we moved Mom to an Adult Family Home, my sister was very involved with shopping and preparing meals. After moving Mom to the Adult Family Home, both my sister and I felt guilty that we did not take her into our homes. We discussed the pros/cons and answer was always the same: Mom is too difficult for us to handle. Sometimes I think I was just being selfish, not wanting to interrupt my life. Mostly, I know that I could not have handled her. Helen's daughter, OR

~ After Mom was place in the Adult Family Home, I was relieved that she was in a safe environment and that they attempted to feed her a decent diet. However, the medical problems continued and she seemed angry and combative about being at the home. She said [about my sister and me], "They dumped me here and took all my money." Helen's daughter, WA

~ We went home frequently and called frequently. While in Superior, I would try to set up services such as Meals-on-Wheels, rides to church, etc. All suggestions were met with hostility. Mother insisted she would not leave her home. My aunt and uncle felt we were negligent; we felt she had enough help to keep her safe but felt guilty as not all agreed with us. Mary's stepdaughter, MN

~ My day did center around Mom. Mornings, I'd get Mom up by 8 a.m.; I had her cereal and meds ready. Next, I put her in the shower and laid her clothes out. After a little help like drying her toes and finishing dressing, I had her on the bus [to adult daycare] by 9:20 or sitting in the living room where she liked watching people pass. Myra's daughter, MN

~ I got many phone calls from Mom (Dad dialed for her) expressing her unhappiness and paranoia. She complained constantly about Dad and the helper. She moved things around all the time; it was a nightmare to find things Mildred's daughter, IA

~ About this time, I heard of a support group in Des Moines. They met twice a month and this is where I met "Gerald's wife, IA". I had a 45 mile drive each way but it was worth it. I would have these strange thoughts about "why" and "death" and many others that I didn't think I should be having. By sharing them with other caregivers, I found out that they weren't so out of line as I had thought. If I had discussed them with someone that wasn't familiar with AD, they would have thought I had really gone off the deep end. We tell people in our group now that feelings are OK and need to be shared in the group. We call ourselves "married singles" and don't seem to fit anywhere. We do a lot of laughing at our meetings, much better than crying. The group always recommended that we look around for a nursing home before we need one – very hard to do. Reatha's husband, IA

~ Carol misplaced her rings a couple of times; we now have a place to put them. She does not like to answer the phone when it rings so I now have a cell phone that picks up our home phone number. Carol's husband, MN

~ My sister was the primary caregiver. She received many calls from Mom to come RIGHT NOW because she "couldn't walk" or was feeling sick. My sister finally had to weigh each call before rushing to Mom's side. My sister lived 26 miles from Mom and the calls during the night were the worst. We finally had the nursing home unplug her phone at night because if she didn't feel the staff or my sister were coming fast enough, she would dial 9-1-1. Matilda's daughter, MN

~ I had "my life" only when Gerald was at day care: library, doctor, grocery store, bank, etc., sewing name tags on his clothing. When he was home, he followed me to every room. He didn't want me to talk on the telephone. I had to watch him every minute to keep him safe. It was maddening to answer the same questions all day long. It was difficult not to get angry, not to run away myself. Gerald's wife, IA

~ Dad did continue to golf early on. We probably should not have let him go as we realize now that he had gotten lost several times. The golfers were good to him and helped him a lot. Alvin's daughter, IA

~ Mom had to adjust to Dad being around more and eventually had to do more and more for him. She was careful about moving things of his to prevent him from being angered when he could not find something. Also friction between them increased some, occasionally, due to his constant presence where it had not previously existed. Joe's daughter, IA

~ The calls regarding a lost purse or billfold increased and there was no calm until I had left work to go to her house to find the lost item. I was more aware of needing to be vigilant in all things but really didn't know the reality of what the future eventually would bring. I called her more often. I worried about money for her care down the road.   Lanie's daughter, MN

YOUR THOUGHTS -

_____

_____

_____

_____

_____

_____

_____

_____

_____

_____

_____

_____

_____

_____

Even an angel can't do two things at the same time. (Midrash: *Genesis Rabbah* 50:2)

The driving dilemma

~ This was easy for us as Mom hit a post while attempting to park the car and turned in her car keys to my sister. The car was in Mom's garage but she never drove it again. She was happy to still have the car and my sister used it to take Mom everywhere she needed to go.   Matilda's daughter, MN

~ Driving was the big monster. Finally, I would just refuse to ride with him. He would finally let me drive. Our car had two keys (one ignition only; the other for the doors only). I took the ignition key off his key ring. When he couldn't start the car, I would say, "Scoot over, let me try my key." When I was driving, he constantly criticized me: too fast, should have turned, do I know where I'm going, etc., etc. A real nightmare.   Gerald's wife, IA

~ The physician scheduled tests (cognitive) to tell us where Dad was at with capabilities to drive. Dad failed them. He cannot understand why he cannot drive any longer. He argues with me and others that he is fine and that others who are driving should not be. We've not sold his car and try to take him out in it occasionally.   Roy's daughter, MN

~ One day I was driving behind her on a very busy highway and she had a left turn signal [arrow] that was red. She went right through it and I shut my eyes and prayed for the best. There was a lot of horn-honking but she made it. Another time, she was following me on that same busy road and the light changed to red just as I got through the intersection. She went right through the red light.   Lanie's sister, MN

~ My mother did not drive. When I retired, part of her social security went toward car upkeep. She always liked to go for a drive.   Marie's daughter, MN

~ Mom hid the car keys so Dad couldn't find them. That took care of his driving.   Alvin's daughter, IA

~ Mom's primary-care doctor told her he did not want her driving any more. He based this on the evaluation and our input. She was devastated but cooperated in selling her car. Now Mom says she is "trapped" and has lost all of her independence. She is very angry about it and feels she is capable of driving since she doesn't go on the freeways anyway. Story: Mom got into the car at one point to drive us somewhere and said, "Let's see. I'm going backward – that's the 'R', right?"
                                                                                                                  Ann's daughter, MN

~ Clarence didn't want to drive the car for two years before his death; he asked me to do the driving. He took his drivers license out of his pocketbook [billfold].
Clarence's wife, SC

~ Carol is still doing some driving although it is for only a very short distance. She is very aware of going somewhere that she does not remember well. Just before she was diagnosed with AD, she was going to sit with the grandchildren at our daughter's home about 20 miles away but got lost and arrived there about four hours later. Since that time, she does not go more than a mile from home by herself. I watch this very closely but don't want to restrict at this stage.
Carol's husband, MN

~ We let Mother drive much too long. She would get lost driving to familiar places or lose her car in parking ramps and insist it was stolen. Finally, my brother came home and took the car. She never got over the fact that Tom came and stole her car!
Mary's stepdaughter, MN

~ Mother tried to drive but fortunately I said "wouldn't it be nice to have a chauffeur" and she sort of went along with it. When the doctor told her to put the keys away for good, she became very upset and said she had been driving since she was 12 years old. The doctor urged her to stop before she had an accident. She then told everyone that I made her stop driving and that I was the one that had pushed it on the doctor to tell her not to drive.
Charlotte's daughter, TX

~ We had to take Mom's car away when she started getting lost going to my youngest sister's house. Mom would then try to go back to her original apartment instead of the assisted living place. We had a doctor instruct us to not let her drive any more which made it easier for us (my younger sister). Mom was mad at us for a long time about that.
Donna's daughter, IA

~ That one was pretty easy. Mom pretty much decided that driving was too scary. At one point, she asked me to be with her when she drove and she became confused. That was pretty much the end of the issue. Shortly after that, we made the decision to move her because the burden on my sister to run Mom's errands was just too much, plus we knew it would just get worse. To my mother's credit, she did eventually recognize that she should not drive. She was scared of getting lost after driving around for quite some time, a trauma she apparently remembered quite well.
Helen's daughter, OR

~ I did not take Mom's car away when I should have because I was avoiding the fight – this was my biggest "ostrich moment" (as in head in the sand so I didn't have to deal with the issue) regarding the disease. Luckily, she didn't have an accident or anything – just often couldn't remember how to put the car in gear or turn it off. We argued about the car **a lot**. I finally called the MN Department of Transportation for help and they suggested I "turn her in" anonymously as a driver that should be retested. When she got the letter from the DOT about coming in to discuss her driving, she hid it from me (but I had been copied on it). She had such a strong regard for authority, she did let me put her car "in storage" after that. Thinking about it later, I acknowledged that she could have been in an accident and hurt or killed someone and she wouldn't even have remembered it! I would have had to live with it, though. We were very lucky.   Lanie's daughter, MN

YOUR THOUGHTS -

_____

_____

_____

_____

_____

_____

_____

_____

_____

_____

It's good to hope but bad to depend on it. (proverb)

The comfort of familiar things

~ She took care of her plants, did the wash, bathed herself and talked to her sister a lot on the phone. I think in the first 1-2 years, she did some baking but think she was more than ready to leave it all up to me. Marie's daughter, MN

~ Mom and Dad lived in an apartment after they retired from farming. As the disease progressed, they moved to a retirement home which helped Mom because they served 1 meal there. If Mom was there, Dad was happy. Alvin's daughter, IA

~ Alvin continued to carry his Bible and devotion book around with him although he never read a word. I never argued with him on anything. Alvin didn't like to be without me around. Alvin's wife, IA

~ He did not want the home furnishings moved around and insisted on the same daily routines (up and down at same times, mealtimes, etc.) Joe's wife, IA

~ Mom liked to read a lot and play cribbage. She did not have many things from her home in Tucson. She did have a favorite loveseat and TV which we moved to our house. She was very good at needlepoint which she did a lot of. Milta's son, KS

~ Mother had a cat called "Lisa" she dearly loved. She also had a subscription to the *National Enquirer* which she believed every word. She loved garage sales and bought things if they were under $1 (but 25¢ was the best!). She had so much stuff but then we would recycle items so she would have room for more. So why not give her pleasure? Margaret's daughter, KS

~ Sometimes, Gerald played solitaire almost all day. We would take walks most every day. He "read" large print western books; usually fell asleep. TV was confusing to him. That was the time of the O. J. Simpson trial and every time the trial was mentioned, it was all new to him. Gerald liked to help me by doing the dishes. (It was like "hide-and-seek" to find things sometimes.) Gerald's wife, IA

~ Dad feeds the birds and squirrels and enjoys watching them eat from the window in their living room. He still attempts to do things in a routine. He forgets so much that if he re-does something or questions us for an appointment or day or whatever, he is unaware of the time lapse and that he just asked that, and goes on about the day without the awareness of having just done something. Roy's daughter, MN

~ I would often take her on rides to places we visited as children, including the house we lived in well into our teens. The church we attended had not changed at all and she lit up when she saw it. *Lanie's sister, MN*

~ Clarence loved the cat we got in May 2003 and the cat loved him. He finally got so he didn't want to read the morning newspaper. He told me to tell him if there was anything he should know. *Clarence's wife, SC*

~ Mom liked to play cards and that is the one thing she enjoyed doing at her assisted living quarters but she often said she had nothing to do because she wouldn't remember having played. She still liked to go to the casino and knew what to do when she got there. *Donna's daughter, IA*

~ I contacted a parish member to pick Mom up for daily Mass (a part of Mom's routine for years). In her apartment, she is surrounded by all of her furniture, pictures, etc. from her house. She continues to cross-stitch, read and go for walks and occasionally socializes with old friends. *Ann's daughter, MN*

~ Reatha and I would continue doing what we always had done, doing quite a bit of walking, holding hands and going out to Burger King for supper. One night, while we were in line, she started eating french fries from the tray a man was carrying behind us. I explained the situation and he was very nice about it. *Reatha's husband, IA*

~ Mom took pride in still writing checks while I sat with her. She wanted to keep as independent as possible. She subscribed to the *Journal* [local paper] but never read it anymore. I'd pick out an article and try to get conversation going. Mom always checked her calendar each day to make sure she <u>would not</u> miss her hair appointment *Myra's daughter, MN*

~ Carol enjoys going to church and our couples Bible study group although she just listens. She enjoys our older grandchildren (teenagers and older) but becomes very edgy around young children with their play. She likes getting the daily paper and reads all the ads in the Sunday paper. *Carol's husband, MN*

~ My Mom's purse – she always had to know where it was. At the nursing home, I gave her a cosmetic bag with a few dollars, some change and a comb inside. She thought it was her purse and seemed comforted about knowing it was in the drawer of her bedside table. *Genevieve's daughter, MN*

~ Mom took great pride in feeding the neighborhood's stray cats and continued to do that until she moved to her apartment. Until she needed to go into the nursing home, she always read the morning paper completely through – that was her morning ritual. She had subscriptions to *Star* and the *National Enquirer* tabloids and thoroughly read those, too. She also continued to go to the casino. Until the very end, she responded to babies and children. Mom recognized her great-grandson, Riley, as someone to fuss over in a grandmotherly way.   Lanie's daughter, MN

YOUR THOUGHTS -

If you can't do what you want, do what you can. (proverb)

Dealing with the forgetfulness

~ It was like a 33 rpm record stuck in a groove playing the same song phrase over and over. During a visit or a phone conversation, Mom would repeat the same story multiple times and clearly not know she had already told me. For me this was fine; I understood. As time went on, a smaller set of stories from earlier periods in time (younger ages) were being retold. Eventually, she asked where her parents were and wanted to go home (even though she was now at her own home). Clearly, she wanted to go to her childhood home. I surely hope this means that she remembered in some fashion that she felt safe and cared for in that childhood family home.   Helen's daughter, OR

~ When driving Mom somewhere, she would ask every five minutes, "Where are we going and what are we going to do there?"   Helen's daughter, WA

~ After a while, Mom wouldn't remember what we were doing or where we were going.   Donna's daughter, IA

~ The forgetfulness mainly manifested in hallucinations ("dancing kittens") and in failure to recognize family members. Grandma looked at me and said, "Oh, you're Miss USA!" My polo shirt had "USA" embroidered on it. (I'd never actually been "Miss USA" prior to that moment – the humor in this actually comforts me.)   Gen's granddaughter, CA

~ Mom has notes in several places. So far, she takes care of her apartment and is well-groomed (she continues to have her hair done once a week). The forgetfulness is more and more apparent. She forgets her grandchildren's names, could not think of the word "Band-Aid", makes grocery lists with odd names (i.e. "facell tissues" for "Kleenex"), asked where the stamp goes on a letter.   Ann's daughter, MN

~ For the last two years in Mom's life, she never remembered who I was. Sometimes, I was Irene, her sister. She often talked about Joan, my sister, but I was lost in that fog of her mind. Although I mentioned who I was daily, she just knew a lady had come to give her meds, change and washing things for her and bring sweets.   Myra's daughter, MN

~ Carol spends a lot of time worrying about the prescriptions that she is taking: thinking that she may forget to take one, asks questions. If they are repetitive, I write down the question and answer for her on a piece of paper. This helps me and eases her concerns.   Carol's husband, MN

~ I remember weekends at the cabin: most of our time was spent hunting for her purse.   Mary's stepdaughter, MN

~ My Mom will start to say a sentence and halfway through, forget what she wanted to say or even the subject. I now finish sentences for her and that she tolerates well. Mother forgets the days of the week. She can no longer tell time on her own watch: she will say it is 9 a.m. when it is 8 a.m. Charlotte's daughter, TX

~ If Mom went to a club meeting, we could expect a call from Dad asking where Mom was not more than ten minutes after she left. Alvin's daughter, IA

~ Short-term memory got worse as the months with us passed. Had a hard time keeping track of where she was in cribbage and needlepoint. One bright spot was reading. She loved Erma Bombeck and read and laughed at the same book over and over. She couldn't remember that she had read it so it was always new. Milta's son, KS

~ Mother always asked new people if they had ever been to Minnesota or if they had been on a farm. Margaret's daughter, KS

~ Mom's endless questions and constant repeating often left us completely drained after a visit with her. Most of her questions had to do with people she knew back in the 1930s, making it hard for us to answer. Mary's daughter, MN

~ I took care of his medicines. I would remind him to shower and laid out his clothes, taking away others. He seemed content for me to be "in charge". He would forget he just ate and would want to eat. He couldn't tell time. Mostly, I remember his doing what I would tell him. Gerald's wife, IA

~ Dad asks the same questions over and over, as if he is caught in a loop. I call to remind him when I am on my way to pick him up for an outing or appointments. Often, I will start reminding him the night before an outing. This will assist him in at least knowing that he is going out the next day. This can backfire sometimes; he will call early in the morning, wondering why I am late and I will explain that I am not late – he is just early! Roy's daughter, MN

~ Joe got to where he did not want to shower and/or change his clothes. Joe's wife, IA

~ My mother would ask many of the same questions over and over. She would never miss church so I would tell her "It's Sunday" and pick out her clothes. She always knew what she was doing in church for 1-2 years. Marie's daughter, MN

~ We all learned to just listen every time she repeated things. Matilda's daughter, MN

~ Like most AD patients, Mom could endlessly repeat questions because she quickly forgot the answer. She had a hard time remembering that we had plans for dinner or an outing unless I called her immediately prior to picking her up. As mentioned previously, her purse was often "lost" somewhere in the house. She did remember to bathe but taking care of her beautiful hair was not part of her routine.

Lanie's daughter, MN

YOUR THOUGHTS -

_____

_____

_____

_____

_____

_____

_____

_____

_____

_____

_____

_____

_____

> **Humor is an affirmation of dignity, a declaration of man's superiority to all that befalls him.**
>
> (Romain Gary, *Promise at Dawn*)

_____

_____

_____

_____

_____

_____

_____

_____

_____

_____

_____

_____

_____

Scary incidents and their outcomes

~ Being in the car with Joe when he forgot where we were going or where we were. Joe's wife, IA

~ At one point, when Dad still drove the car, he turned the ignition off as he approached the drive (like he used to do many years ago with a straight stick [transmission]) to coast into the drive, only to find that he had no power steering and no power brakes. He hit the house, breaking siding and the basement wall and damaging his pickup. Joe's daughter, IA

~ Mom had a serious nosebleed and had to go to Emergency to have a packing. When home, she would forget what it was for and pull it out of her nose and start the bleeding again. Had to have her in the hospital, restrained for several days to heal. She got real mad at that. Milta's son, KS

~ Mother liked to go to garage sales and she would walk (this is when she first moved from MN) to K-Mart which was a good mile away. The clerk would call and we would pick her up. One time, she walked further and a policeman offered to take her home but she said, "My daughter would get very upset if I came home in a police car!!" Margaret's daughter, KS

~ In the assisted living place, Mom had three fires. This was due to the fact that she made toast in the oven and would sit down for a short nap and forget everything. She did have a toaster. Due to this, her stove was shut off. Mary's daughter, MN

~ Mom's vision was very bad. She would turn on the stove or start the oven only to call someone to come because the stove wasn't working. The stove worked but she couldn't see the dials. Matilda's daughter, MN

~ Gerald would get up in the middle of the night, agitated, setting off our security alarm. He'd hear noises and people and telephones. He'd turn on lights. He'd insist I get ready to go someplace with him. Gerald's wife, IA

~ Early in the disease, I spent the night with Grandma in her apartment. She didn't sleep for more than 10 minutes at any time. She talked to long-deceased relatives as if they were in her room. At one point, I lined dining room chairs around her bed to try to keep her in bed. While I was lying on the floor by her bedroom door, I heard her say "I'd like to get up, too, but I think it would make that lady out there mad." Gen's granddaughter, CA

~ Falls – at the apartment – leaving the stove burners on and burning pans – leaving her patio door open all night – losing keys (over and over again). Thank God, nothing terrible happened at the apartment through all this. Genevieve's daughter, MN

~ One Saturday, my husband and I came with a few groceries. Upon opening the door, the smell of gas was extremely bad. A burner was turned on but no flame. We both flew around opening windows and both doors. Mom just smiled. We disconnected the stove right then.   Myra's daughter, MN

~ Once mother was driving to St. Paul for a graduation party. She gave me a call and said, "I'm at the mall." She didn't know what mall. I had her put down the phone and ask what mall she was at. She did this and I found her. Another time, I went to the St. Paul Amtrak depot to meet Mom [who had had been put on the train by my cousins in Superior, WI]. When she didn't get off the train, I talked to the conductor and he said that a lady had gotten off in Sandstone, claiming she wanted to get to Superior. I knew the Sandstone "depot" is in a drugstore so I called them and they said a woman had been there all morning. I asked them to keep her and I raced to Sandstone [a distance of about 80 miles].   Mary's stepdaughter, MN

~ Last fall, I was helping Dad while he was parking his riding lawn mower. He rammed it into another piece of equipment. He would back the lawn mower up and try to park it again, again hitting another piece of equipment. I began to realize that all of his faculties were no longer there.   Roy's daughter, MN

~ I had a similar experience as my niece with Lanie's gas stove. I walked into a gas-filled house and went to Lanie's stove. The burner was on but the pilot light was out. I called the gas company and we stayed outside until they checked the whole house for gas leaks. If I hadn't been there to pick Lanie up, I'm sure she would have died.   Lanie's sister, MN

~ Stove burner left on under the teapot and burned it; keys locked in car with car running.   Ann's daughter, MN

~ Fortunately, we did not have any big/scary incidents, I believe mainly because my sister kept close watch/contact with Mom. My sister did describe Mom calling her saying that she had nothing to eat – what should she do? After talking Mom through looking in the pantry to see what was there, it was clear to my sister that we were in trouble and had to make some changes. That is when the challenges really began – what were those changes?   Helen's daughter, OR

~ On a weekend when my sister stayed with my Mom, my sister accidentally forgot her luggage at my Mom's place. Mom was frantic about the "unknown bag" and thought a stranger had been in her home. She wanted me to call the police.   Helen's daughter, WA

~ Once, when still in her house, the pilot light on one of Mom's gas stove's burners went out. Because Mom had lost her sense of smell, she didn't know it. For some reason, I dropped by to see her and was almost overwhelmed by the gas odor when I walked in the door. She was at a loss as to why I was racing around opening windows and making her go out on the front porch. The other pilot lights could have ignited the fumes at any time — it was a near thing.   Lanie's daughter, MN

YOUR THOUGHTS -

_____

_____

_____

_____

_____

_____

_____

_____

_____

_____

_____

_____

When a parent helps a child, both smile:
when a child must help a parent, both cry
(variation on a proverb)

_____

_____

_____

_____

_____

_____

_____

_____

_____

_____

_____

_____

_____

_____

_____

_____

Wandering and other potentially dangerous behavior

~ One morning, Gerald took the car by himself while I was in a back bedroom ironing. I went to the kitchen to see how he was doing playing solitaire and he and the car were gone. We immediately released descriptions to the local authorities so they could keep an eye out for Gerald and the car. That afternoon, he called and asked me where **I** was. He said he was in "Knoxville" but didn't understand about putting more money into the pay phone and we were disconnected. We notified Knoxville, IA authorities right away about this call but they couldn't see the car. At this point, the IA highway patrol was also involved. At 11:00 that night, I got a call from a man in Seneca, KS. He had found our car abandoned at the edge of the highway and a man walking in the ditch, acting as if he was looking for something. The Good Samaritan took Gerald home with him and because Gerald still carried identification at that time, I got this most-welcome call. A "rescue team" started on the 5 hour drive to Seneca immediately. Gerald had driven until he ran out of gas. His reason for going? He said he just wanted to go to the casino (I wouldn't take him).

Gerald's wife, IA

~ Thankfully, Dad hasn't had any episodes of misplacing himself – so far . . . A big part of this is because physically, he cannot go too far. Otherwise, he probably would have had a situation of needing to be rescued. It is still a concern.

Roy's daughter, MN

~ One day I told Lanie that I would take her to the local grocery store to shop. When I came to the last stop sign before her apartment building, I saw her standing at the corner, waiting for the light to change – she had forgotten I was coming to get her. Another time, I went upstairs to get her and she wasn't there. I went downstairs to look around and found her walking around in the recreational area. Scary experiences for me because anything could have happened to her.

Lanie's sister, MN

~ Mom never wandered. One summer day, though, she locked herself out. She sat on the porch and when the neighbor lady came home from work, I got a call.

Myra's daughter, MN

~ Last winter, we sent to Las Vegas on vacation. At one of the large casinos, Carol went to the bathroom. I sat down at a slot machine next to the bathroom door but she went out of another door thinking it was the way she went in. I finally had to get security to help me find her. When we met up, she said, "Let's go – this place is too large for me to be in." I don't know who was more upset.

Carol's husband, MN

~ Mom was so afraid, she never wandered.   Mary's daughter, MN

~ Mom got lost in the grocery store, couldn't remember where the bathroom was at my house and had to wear an alarm at the nursing home when she wandered out and off the campus, trying to take the bus to see "Mae" (her cousin).
Genevieve's daughter, MN

~ During one incident, the police brought her home. She was on her way to Mass, walking down the middle of the street in January.   Mary's stepdaughter, MN

~ My Mom is nearly afraid of her own shadow. She has not wandered yet. However, she had stepped off of the front porch and fallen. Luckily, again so far – no broken bones. I sleep with my bedroom door open. I can hear every move she makes. Our home is very small. I would know if she got up in the middle of the night.   Charlotte's daughter, TX

~ Dad tended to roam, especially at night. Mom put a hook on the door that Dad did not realize was there.
Alvin's daughter, IA

~ I would walk her around the block or, if she insisted on going alone, I'd go outside and watch her. Margaret's daughter, KS

~ Mom wandered out of the house twice in the middle of the night. Dad was deaf when his hearing aids were out. The village cop brought her home both times. She was pretty scratched up and cold each time. This precipitated her admission to a nursing home. I suggested better door locks but Dad was pretty well worn out by this time and insisted she be admitted. There were also many badly burned pans and skillets in the house.   Mildred's daughter, IA

~ One of the reasons we placed Grandma in a care facility was fear that she would wander from one of our homes – the guilt would have been awful. Because my parents' home has many stairs, I worried that Grandma's unfamiliarity of environment combined with confusion could result in a serious fall.   Gen's granddaughter, CA

~ Contrary to traditional AD behavior, we had no wandering issues.   Helen's daughter, OR

~ Mom was afraid to go out of the house by herself when she lived there and stuck pretty close to her apartment, too. The one major wandering incident she did have at the apartment resulted in her being evicted as a security risk. She got up in the middle of the night because she said she smelled gas, took the elevator downstairs and said that someone hit her in the stomach. She was so frightened. Because it was a "secure" building, they were afraid she would let someone in during the night if she wandered again. Her eviction required that I quickly find other housing and, at that point, I knew it would be in a nursing home. I couldn't take the chance that there would be another wandering episode and something would happen to her.

Lanie's daughter, MN

YOUR THOUGHTS -

_____

_____

_____

_____

_____

_____

_____

_____

_____

_____

_____

Oh that I had wings like a dove!
For then I would fly away, and be at rest.

(Bible, *Psalms 55:6*)

Exhibiting obsessive behavior

~ Wandering around the house aimlessly, sitting down, standing up, looking at photo albums, putting them down, opening the front door and closing it only to do it again in a couple of minutes, stomping her feet over and over, pounding her cane on the floor over and over, yelling "shut up" or "stop that" for seemingly no reason, yelling at the TV when she seemed to not like what was on, swearing ("bull---t") from time to time for no apparent reason (although usually she was staring at the TV at the time), getting her coat and asking when we were leaving. For a period of several months, she wanted to out in the car. On one day, we went out four different times for a total of 125 miles! Eventually, though, she did not want to go anywhere or do anything.
Helen's daughter, OR

~ Mom always counted her money when we took her to the casino – a ten minute drive. She would count it, put it back, close her purse and then start over. She did this until we arrived and then would say, "Do I have any cash with me?"
Donna's daughter, IA

~ Mom had to touch, feel, discuss and question every solitary item that was in her house as we tried to move her. She was obsessively attached to material objects of no worth or use.
Ann's daughter, MN

~ Mom was always moving her clothes around between two closets. Also, the purse or her cane tended to "disappear" but we were always able to find them.
Myra's daughter, MN

~ "Where is my purse?" was always being asked. Having enough milk in the refrigerator was an obsession as well – and bread. She would keep getting those things until I caught on to take inventory before shopping.
Genevieve's daughter, MN

~ Mother's purse was always missing. She did accuse people of stealing from her because she misplaced so many things.
Mary's stepdaughter, MN

~ Some days, my Mom will tell me over and over again something we need – like, "Get butter at the store." She repeats herself a lot.
Charlotte's daughter, TX

~ I can only recall the multiple calls about losing/misplacing the kids (her great-grandchildren) she thought she was babysitting. They were never actually there.
Gen's granddaughter, CA

~ At about 4:00 p.m. daily, Dad would move all the furniture to the middle of the room. I don't know why. Alvin's daughter, IA

~ Alvin moved the furniture to the middle of the room. Nobody knew why. He worried about the "cattle" that were out. Actually, they were bushes.   Alvin's wife, IA

~ When she was still at home, Mom had to know where Dad was at all times. She became very agitated when he went for the mail or to the farm. Unrealistic in her time expectations.   Mildred's daughter, IA

~ Mother seemed to be very fearful and very protective of her purse. She took it everywhere. In fact, she usually hid it in her bed and slept with it. She always wanted money in her purse but seemed to lose every bit of it. We never were able to find any of the money.   Mary's daughter, MN

~ Whenever Mom felt she needed something for herself or something needed to be done to the house, it had to be done "right now" and she would make calls every half-hour asking, "When are you coming?"   Matilda's daughter, MN

~ Gerald was obsessed with his billfold. He spent hours going through the billfold, taking out each card, counting the money, putting everything back, taking it all out again, hour after hour, over and over. And he was obsessed with his keys - he had always carried lots of keys.   Gerald's wife, IA

~ Dad is a recovered alcoholic but insists on drinking non-alcoholic beer. If he is getting low, he will call or tell me over and over that he needs his beer. Previously, his obsession has been vitamins. He spent a lot of money on them. I recently cleaned out his vitamin cabinet and disposed of three full bags because the vitamins had expired. And last, but not least, Dad has a health issue regularly – hypochondria? A sister who is a nurse suggested telling him less about his medical stuff – otherwise, he will overreact.   Roy's daughter, MN

~ She would get very angry at some of the other residents at the nursing home and would actually hit them. This behavior from a person who wouldn't swat a fly was very upsetting. Her purse was her biggest object of obsession. Even in the nursing home, she had to have it in the "pocket" of the walker.   Lanie's sister, MN

~ Again, the purse comes to mind. She had to be able to see it and touch it in order to be calm. As Mom got worse (but was still living independently), she continued to get her newspapers and tabloids but couldn't keep up. She'd stack them up "to read later" and wouldn't allow me to get rid of them. I'd also consider going to the casinos to be obsessive behavior as she did not understand the possible consequences of her gambling, but she still went regularly.   Lanie's daughter, MN

YOUR THOUGHTS -

_____

_____

_____

_____

_____

_____

_____

_____

_____

_____

_____

_____

Handling money and legal matters

~ My mother was always in charge of her checkbook and balanced her bank statement. I found unpaid bills or checks missing. At first, she was "so sure" she could do this that I would have to sneak paying bills. I believe I let her keep her own register of payments but I had my own and let her do what she wanted. She wasn't aware she was screwing things up.

Marie's daughter, MN

~ When they went shopping or out to eat, Dad would hand his billfold to the clerk and say, "Take what you need." After that happened, Mom would put only $20.00 in his billfold. Mom had Power of Attorney. Alvin's daughter, IA

~ Mom handled her own money even after she went to the nursing home. Once her eyesight got so bad that she couldn't see where to sign her name on the checks, my sister finally took over the bill paying which made Mom quite upset. As her illness became worse, Mom never asked about the bill paying, etc. Matilda's daughter, MN

~ Hardest thing for me: lying to someone I had never lied to in 50 years. And taking money and credit cards out of his billfold (he never realized they were gone). I had always handled the checkbook and paid the bills. I had done the legal papers just in time because now Gerald could no longer sign his name. Gerald's wife, IA

~ My Dad did not take care of the finances; my mother did and still does. Dad is still able to manage a little cash. However, he is so forgetful that we have to show caution with how much he has and to remind him that when he has cash, he has spent it on this or that. Roy's daughter, MN

~ Dad always took care of finances. After he died and she was diagnosed with AD, my brother and I had Power of Attorney. Most of her money was in a trust account handled by a bank trustee in Minneapolis. We were signers on her checking account. Milta's son, KS

~ We had a joint checking account and I took care of all her bills. Margaret's daughter, KS

~ Dad got DPA [Durable Power of Attorney] and Mom no longer wanted to deal with money. Mildred's daughter, IA

~ I did have Power of Attorney for Mom because I was her only survivor. Mary's daughter, MN

70

~ I remember very well Lanie's many trips to the casinos. When I would ask her how she did, she'd say she came back with two or three hundred dollars in her purse. What I didn't know was that it probably cost her five or six hundred to get it. She had always been so in control of her own life so this was a complete shock to me when I found out about her problem. I offered to balance her checkbook once and it was in terrible shape.   Lanie's sister, MN

~ Mom willingly gave POA [Power-of-Attorney] to my sister and me (we are the only children; my father is deceased). Mom is unable to make out checks but can still sign them. She saves all paperwork for my sister to review because Mom can't make sense of most of it.   Ann's daughter, MN

~ Mom accepted the fact she needed help with the checkbook, etc., so my sister Joan and I both had Power of Attorney.
                    Myra's daughter, MN

~ I am in the process of arranging our finances so that everything will not be used for Carol's care with nothing left for my later years. She is very conscious of our finances at this time.   Carol's husband, MN

~ My brother took care of the bills when Mom was unable to do so. Finally, we couldn't <u>find</u> the bills. They would be tucked away in her underwear drawer, etc. The three siblings met with Mom and Brian pretty much forced her to give him Power of Attorney. She was hurt.   Mary's stepdaughter, MN

~ My younger sister did most of Mom's money management – usually had to straighten out Mom's checkbook and pay bills that Mom missed.   Donna's daughter, IA

~ Finances were done by Dad so when he died, Mom was clueless. After his death, I tried to teach her to use the ATM to get cash, but she did not understand. She'd write a check and get the cash at the bank (that's fine) but eventually, my sister and I had to start filling out the check. She never did an ATM transaction: it was always done by me on her behalf. Thankfully, she relied on us daughters to take care of the major items. In the early days, she was still able to pay bills but she received contribution envelopes from her church and thought she should start giving several hundred dollars a month. We realized that perhaps it was time to make a change. We got her to agree to my sister being on the checking account, diverted her mail to my sister and my sister started paying the bills. Problem solved – for a while – until Mom could no longer live at home alone.   Helen's daughter, OR

~ For decades, Mom kept business financial books as part of her job. Her checkbook was always balanced. The disease took away any sense of the value of money and she gambled a lot. Her source of gambling money was cash advances on credit cards that she signed up for as a result of direct mail offers. I did not find out about this until she was deeply in debt (over $100,000) and then only because of a personal banker who bent the rules regarding privacy to show me what Mom was doing. I will bless her forever. I was able to work with Mom to assign me Durable Power of Attorney so I could "speak" for her when it became necessary. I put myself on her checking account as well. I looked into bankruptcy for her but she would have none of that so we put first and second mortgages on Mom's house (which had never had a mortgage) to try and pay off the debt. Ironically, the good credit that got Mom into trouble also let her get mortgages fairly easily. I helped get her a job where I worked so that she could have some income to pay on the mortgages. However, she was only able to work for a relatively short time before her job performance was unacceptable due to the AD progression. At that point, she did have to file for bankruptcy. We had hoped to be able to hang onto the house but her income (pension and Social Security) didn't cover the mortgages. This is when I started the paperwork to move her into public housing. The banks eventually took the house, which my Dad had built with his own hands. This was a very stressful time for me.

Lanie's daughter, MN

YOUR THOUGHTS -

_____

_____

_____

_____

_____

_____

_____

_____

Melancholy creates nervous ailments; cheerfulness cures them. (proverb)

_____
_____
_____
_____
_____
_____
_____
_____
_____
_____
_____
_____
_____
_____
_____
_____

Caring for pets

~ Dad farmed and took care of cattle and he took good care of the cats on the farm. When they moved to town, he had his imaginary cats and cattle that he would need to feed and care for. Alvin's daughter, IA

~ As above re: cats and cattle. I never argued with him that there were no cattle or cats here. Alvin's wife, IA

~ Mother had her cat, "Lisa", and kept her in her room all the time. After Mother passed on, Lisa has become more friendly and has the run of the house. Margaret's daughter, KS

~ We'd had a dog 20 years ago and now Gerald was always looking for it or asking where it was. Gerald's wife, IA

~ My Dad seems to be able to care for his dogs. Sometimes, though, he is so forgetful that I remind him to care for them. On occasion, he forgets to feed them. Because I am at my parents' home pretty much daily, I am able to do this. (The other things, like meds for the pets, I take care of.) Roy's daughter, MN

~ Lanie always had a very deep love for animals and her cat was always taken care of, though we had to keep checking the litter box to be sure it was tolerable. Lanie's sister, MN

~ The cat looked all over for Clarence when he went to the hospital; seemed very sad. Clarence's wife, SC

~ Two years ago, I, along with our son and daughter, purchase a Pomeranian dog from a breeder for Carol's birthday. The dog brought instant joy to Carol's life along with the cat we already had. Carol's husband, MN

~ Mother lost her cat from old age about two years before she was diagnosed. We have our "babies" – dogs and cats – with us here at our house. She loves them all but hasn't a clue of how to take care of them. Charlotte's daughter, TX

~ Mom had no pets – she never cared to have them around. However, she prided herself on her African violets inside the house and her geraniums on the deck in the warm weather. As she declined, the violets and geraniums suffered as well. She would forget to water and feed the plants, she could no longer remember to deadhead them and forget to turn them in the sun so that they always looked lopsided. She no longer took joy in the mini-carnation cut flowers I would bring to her nearly every week. Genevieve's daughter, MN

74

~ Mom continued to take good care of her cat, Essie. Essie went with her from the house to the apartment but couldn't go to the nursing home. I called some no-kill shelters but because Essie was not considered adoptable due to her age and health, they would not take her. The cat was not at all well at that point: I opted to have her put to sleep. Since Essie was so neurotic regarding anyone but Mom, I couldn't take her home even for a few days. My aunt and I literally took Essie from the apartment to the vet's to be euthanized after we'd moved Mom to the nursing home. My aunt and I both cried and cried – this was another sad symbol of how Mom's life had declined. Lanie's daughter, MN

A four-legged friend, a four-legged friend, he'll never let you down. (lyric by J. Brooks)

YOUR THOUGHTS -

_____

_____

_____

_____

_____

_____

_____

_____

_____

_____

Getting support from the medical community

~ In general, I found the medical community to minimize the memory deficit if Grandma happened to have a lucid moment in their office. When she finally, in a doctor's office, couldn't name the President and identified my Mom as "Commander-In-Chief of the Navajo Nation", they admitted Grandma to the hospital. We were then advised this would be 48-72 hours only – we'd have to have a plan for her post-discharge care within that time.   Gen's granddaughter, CA

~ In the early stages, Mom respected her primary doctor's opinion, was pleased to see him and he probably was instrumental in convincing Mom to move to the Adult Family Home. But it seemed as if we (actually, my sister) had to push for the doctor(s) to take an interest, consider treatment/drug options, pursue anti-depressants, do tests and send Mom to specialists. In short, my sister guided Mom's treatment more than the doctor did – sad but true. They seemed to want to treat Mom as "just getting old". After an appointment with a geriatric specialist, the doctor, in fact, said something like, "What do you want me to do – she has Alzheimer's." It was only after my sister pushed (yay, sister) that the doctor prescribed anything and only after further pushing modified the prescription. My impression is that they wanted us to "go away". In our community, it is my opinion that Alzheimer's treatment in the HMO medical field is "a joke". On a bright note, a social worker at the same health organization did take an interest in our situation and lobbied on our behalf to get further treatment considerations. The medical field needs to "get a grip" and help the family as much (or more) than the AD patient. We did not receive any referrals, web-site references or phone numbers [for other resources]. My sister (along with her husband) did the work. Bless their hearts, they are/were the heroes. Unless my sister made it happen, it did not happen. My sister was a true and diligent advocate for Mom.   Helen's daughter, OR

~ Mom wouldn't change doctors. Her family doctor was the one we didn't like. In the end, Mom didn't like him either, but we never knew why.   Donna's daughter, IA

~ I would see that she got her flu shots. Her own doctor treated her fine. My mother's health was good – vision, hearing and she very seldom got colds or flu. She was good at keeping herself clean.   Marie's daughter, MN

~ Alvin's doctor was very cooperative – he told me what would happen.   Alvin's wife, IA

76

~ We had a very understanding M.D. that we could confide our problems in and he would gently make suggestions to Dad that he would accept from Dr. but not us.   Joe's daughter, IA

~ I don't think Mom got the greatest medical care but getting household help was encouraged so her personal care improved.   Mildred's daughter, IA

~ The neurologist was dreadful. He was rude to the aide who brought Mom to appointments. I never felt he was kind or supportive to Mom or us.   Mary's stepdaughter, MN

~ Her doctor kept warning me that decisions for Mom would have to be made by me, her only dependent. This was something I had no desire to do.   Mary's daughter, MN

~ We didn't get much support from the medical community. Mom was in a small town and the doctors weren't very knowledgeable. I tried to get information, but my sister or the doctors weren't happy about my interfering.   Matilda's daughter, MN

~ Our family doctor more or less wrote Gerald off – said there was nothing he could do for Gerald. But, he said I needed to take care of myself and put me on Prozac to keep me from crying all the time. He was always comforting and supportive of me.   Gerald's wife, IA

~ The physician who diagnosed Dad with the AD was open to explaining to us, including Dad, that he has this disease. We continue to see him and he continues to oversee my Dad's health issues.   Roy's daughter, MN

~ Mom's doctor is very compassionate and treats her with great respect. I accompany her to all appointments since she doesn't comprehend or remember his instructions. He is very supportive and knowledgeable. Mom likes him because he spends a lot of time with her and talks about other topics with her.   Ann's daughter, MN

~ Mom's doctor was very up-front about Mom's health and well-being. By September, 2001, he informed us that Mom should not live alone: we should pass on assisted living and rather look into a nursing home facility. This was the most difficult decision I had to make.   Myra's daughter, MN

~ My doctor (a female general practitioner), who had diagnosed Mom's Alzheimer's, was very open in discussing the progression of the disease and what to expect. Mom's "old" doctor had insisted that she needed to stop driving so she would no longer go to him (which was fine because he was really an endocrinologist, not even a general/family practitioner). Mom liked him because he flirted with her.

Lanie's daughter, MN

YOUR THOUGHTS -

_____

_____

_____

_____

_____

_____

_____

_____

_____

_____

_____

_____

Resources used at this point

~ We went to an AD class which was very helpful. Also, the book, *The 36 Hour Day,* is excellent. Margaret's daughter, KS

~ I had worked in social services in a care facility so had some knowledge. We encouraged Dad to go to a caregivers' support group but he was unable to hear much of what was going on and refused to return. Mildred's daughter, IA

~ I have some experience with dementia from my occupation the past 24 years that I would apply at times. Joe's daughter, IA

~ My wife and I attended some caregiving programs here which were also sponsored by our local Alzheimer's Association. Milta's son, KS

~ The [nursing home] began an Alzheimer's group when Mother first moved in. I guess you could say we were charter members. The medical doctors encouraged us in joining this group. Mary's daughter, MN

~ I contacted the Alzheimer's Association in MN and received lots of information. I also joined a support group, which was helpful and supportive. I tried to encourage my sister to go as there was a support group not far from her. I think to this day, my sister is in denial of the real problems Mom was having. Matilda's daughter, MN

~ We had close friends (the "D's") that we golfed with weekly and with whom we often played bridge and ate out. Mrs. D. was diagnosed with AD about a year prior to Gerald's diagnosis. When Mrs. D and Gerald were both in day care, Mr. D. and I would have coffee together at the supermarket and could share our problems and got strength from each other. I also had good support from my church, my pastor and church caregivers. Gerald's wife, IA

~ One of my sisters works on the AD ward in a veteran's nursing home and she is able to direct and suggest things to assist and to guide us through dealing with this disease. Also, the Internet is helpful and the local caregiver programs, too. Roy's daughter, MN

~ I read articles about the disease that helped me to understand it. They enabled me to expect what was coming so the changes were not such a shock. Lanie's sister, MN

~ I purchased several books about the brain and researched nutritional and alternative supplements. We visited a naturopathic clinic Helen's daughter, WA

~ I read *The 36 Hour Day* and have talked with contemporaries dealing with the same problems. My sister and I function as each other's sounding board and support. I used the SeniorLinkage Line and "Familink" as resources for seniors, not necessarily AD. My observation is that there are many seniors with varying degrees of dementia, probably caused by AD but simply undiagnosed. The diagnosis is devastating since there really is no effective treatment.

Ann's daughter, MN

~ I signed up right away with the local Alzheimer's chapter. I did go to some meetings [held in a local care facility] but my Mom did not like watching TV with the other residents while I was in the meetings. She said they were all crazy. Consequently, I do not go to any more meetings. I attended several seminars when she was in the hospital. They were informative.

Charlotte's daughter, TX

~ As an RN, my family often turned to me for advice and guidance. This is OK when it's benign stuff but, in this case, I found it difficult to give the info I knew from experience/education. Because AD is not my professional specialty, I did a lot of research/review via the Internet to "prep" for many family questions as well as inform myself.

Gen's granddaughter, CA

~ I used the Internet to read about AD and newsgroups to grasp other's experiences. The local AD support group was good for learning, discussing, sharing and advising. They also had guest speakers that would talk about relevant/related issues: Power of Attorney, wills, rights, treatments, drugs, facilities, etc. I read books like *The 36 Hour Day* and nutrition/herbal books and researched at the health food store.

Helen's daughter, OR

~ We would have discussions between the three of us (sisters) and share the things we had learned via reading material or informative meetings (one sister is a nurse).

Donna's daughter, IA

~ Our daughter and I regularly attend Alzheimer's support groups. The people at our church are also a great support to Carol and me.

Carol's husband, MN

~ I relied on my daughter [a nurse] for most of the information, advice, support and assistance I needed. In private, I screamed and cried. I was fortunate to have good friends to rely on and they would listen and offer support endlessly. I also read a great deal, questioned the RN's and the social workers at the nursing home. I felt lost – answers seemed to be "out there" but I couldn't get a grasp on them.

Genevieve's daughter, MN

~ I used the Internet extensively to try to learn more about the disease. I wanted to know what I could DO about the disease (not much!) and what to expect down the road. I also attended a series of Caregiver programs sponsored by the local chapter of the Alzheimer's Association. I started to pay attention to the research aspect of AD (and still do). One of my dearest friends was also dealing with AD with her Mom, so we could compare notes and be sad together. Lanie's daughter, MN

YOUR THOUGHTS -

_____

_____

_____

_____

_____

_____

_____

_____

_____

_____

_____

_____

Ask advice wherever you will but act according to your own judgment. (proverb)

Extra journaling pages

AUTUMN – The Steady Decline

Family responses and input on decisions

~ My brother lived up north in Bemidji. We stopped going up there. He would call occasionally and talk to her. It was OK to talk if you didn't ask questions – the answers were usually off the mark. My sister came once a week or we went there so Mom did not talk on the phone as much. At this time, her two sisters were showing symptoms.   Marie's daughter, MN

~ My sister and I told Mom whenever it got too much for her, we were willing to place Dad in a care facility. One morning Mom called and said she'd "had enough". We went immediately and found a nursing home with an area especially for AD patients. That was nice as they were specially trained to care for them.   Alvin's daughter, IA

~ Fortunately, all 3 kids are close and able to help make decisions.   Joe's wife, IA

~ We had 4 opinions and sometimes 4 decisions – not always agreeing!   Joe's daughter, IA

~ My brother and I talked often about Mom's problem. He came to KC a couple of times. Both visits were for her medical problems – nosebleed and heart. She had congestive heart problems which she actually died from. Milta's son, KS

~ Dad made most of the decisions and wasn't willing to listen to many suggestions. Before they got home help, my husband and I were going [to Nebraska] once a month and working the whole weekend. My sister-in-law helped with the business only. I bought all the clothes for both.   Mildred's daughter, IA

~ My sister was in total denial of Mom's illness. Her husband wasn't very supportive, either, and often said, "Your Mom is just using you so don't go to her as often as you do." My husband was supportive of my going to visit Mom but was working where it was difficult to take time off, so I most often went by myself. Two of Mom's grandchildren lived close and two were in other states. My nephew felt like his Dad: "don't go so much".   Matilda's daughter, MN

~ I told the family at Thanksgiving (two daughters and spouses; two grandchildren). They were supportive of whatever I wanted to do but the decisions were all mine.   Gerald's wife, IA

~ My sisters have assisted with help and giving time on occasion when they are able to. My mother is still living with Dad but she herself needs care. My husband helps out a lot and even my daughter will contribute to help. On occasion, my brothers will help, too.   Roy's daughter, MN

~ My niece was really the main decision-maker. I am a wimp when it comes to things like this and she always made the choices that would benefit her mom. We did discuss them but she made the final decision. My other sister was rarely available for input because she had a husband and a very busy life. In the summers [when they were in MN], my sister would visit Lanie once or twice a week in the nursing home. Lanie's sister, MN

~ There is just my sister, Joan, and myself in the family. Because Joan is handicapped, all of the personal care, decision-making and handling financial details for Mom were up to me. While I always talked things out with Joan, I felt pressure on how I was handling situations. There was a lot of daily reporting to Joan and extra questions. At times, this was the exhausting part for me. My husband always backed me up. He chauffeured Mom and me for groceries, doctor appointments, church, etc. He never complained. My children were supportive, too. Myra's daughter, MN

~ Our son and daughter have been great in helping out so I can get some time for myself such as weekend retreats with our church. Carol's sisters help by taking her shopping most every Saturday. Carol's husband, MN

~ I feel fortunate that my entire family viewed Grandma as our treasured Matriarch. Aside from me, all my siblings and parents lived near Grandma. Many of my consultations were via phone, but I also made several trips back to Minnesota when necessary. My family was able to meet, to make decisions with Grandma's wishes in mind, and support each other in our decision. Gen's granddaughter, CA

~ I relied heavily on my daughter who is an RN. I feel so fortunate to have had a marvelous support group to question, cry and pray with and sometimes just sit and hold their hand. My four daughters and son would be there immediately if I asked. My husband – who loved my Mom like his own – was there every step of the way. (Years ago, his mother also died of AD after many years in a nursing home.) Our three grandchildren visited regularly and would draw pictures that my mother would have treasured if she were of sound mind. Genevieve's daughter, MN

~ There are five children in the family. Decisions were made and caregiving was done by the three of us in St. Paul. We were able to discuss, cooperate, and agree in nearly all areas. Mary's stepdaughter, MN

~ My sister visited Mom for a couple of days every 6-8 weeks. My daughter visited about once a month. All care decisions were my responsibility. Helen's daughter, WA

~ My aunt, Mom's sister, was very involved in helping with Mom. Mom's other sister was not available except in the summer. My son was in the Army and stationed out of the U.S. so didn't get to see his Nana very often. My daughter did go see her when she could and was a great resource to me with her background in Speech Therapy as Mom declined. All decisions that were made regarding Mom's care were mine.

Lanie's daughter, MN

YOUR THOUGHTS -

_____

_____

_____

_____

_____

_____

_____

_____

_____

_____

_____

_____

_____

_____

Whether you do little or much, let it be out of good intentions. (Talmud; *Shebu'oth*, 15b)

_____

_____

_____

_____

_____

_____

_____

_____

_____

_____

_____

_____

_____

_____

_____

_____

Language challenges

~ Dad would not retrieve the words he wanted and would become very aggravated when trying to explain himself. We would try to guess at what he wanted but we were usually wrong, adding to his distress.　　　Joe's daughter, IA

~ Mother did not have a speech problem but, after a conversation got going, she liked to listen.　　　Margaret's daughter, KS

~ Mom had trouble finding the right words initially and the last 4 years only spoke nonsense or "chanted" what sounded like an [Native American] Indian chant.　　　Mildred's daughter, IA

~ Part of Mother's problems was the necessity for her to wear two hearing aids. She really didn't like them and was constantly adjusting them.　　　Mary's daughter, MN

~ Mom's speech was not a problem until the last two weeks of her life. We were never able to understand what she was saying and don't know for sure that she understood us although sometimes she would smile at a joke we told.
Matilda's daughter, MN

~ Gerald's speech changed to gibberish: fragmented sentences and nonsense. I observed patients that still responded with "please" and "thank you" for a long time. Gerald could join in the Lord's Prayer for a long time and knew his Social Security number!!　　　Gerald's wife, IA

~ We are pretty certain Dad needs a hearing aid but he refuses.　　　Roy's daughter, MN

~ Lanie was mostly good with her speech until the last couple of months; after that she would just mumble. When we talked to her, she would watch our faces very carefully but could not seem to comprehend what we were saying. Lanie's sister, MN

~ Clarence was hard-of-hearing but refused to wear his hearing aids. His speech was good up until about two months before passing.　　　Clarence's wife, SC

~ Carol's speech is fine at this point. She did get hearing aids about two years ago but only uses them when we go out in public and I insist that she wear them.　　　Carol's husband, MN

~ I have been very satisfied with her care there [in the nursing home]. Reatha started to forget who I was a couple years after placing her there. I became a friend who she would recognize, but not a husband. She began to talk less and now she just jabbers away with very few words that you can recognize. She still is physically strong and could go on several more years. My love for her has never wavered.

Reatha's husband, IA

~ The last eight months, Mom did little talking. I feel placing her in the nursing home sped up the confusion in her mind. I'm glad I managed to keep her in familiar surroundings that extra year. She loved her little green house.

Myra's daughter, MN

~ I was amazed that my Mom's language skills remained pretty much intact. She sometimes couldn't think of a certain word, but she managed quite well overall. Toward the end, she spoke less and less and her voice weakened to the point it was difficult to hear her at times.

Genevieve's daughter, MN

~ For a while, Mom had trouble finding the right words. She spoke less and less and I don't think she spoke at all the last four years of her life.

Mary's stepdaughter, MN

~ My Mom still speaks clearly. However, she has a hearing loss but will not wear hearing aids.

Charlotte's daughter, TX

~ Even though Grandma's memory was rapidly failing, her speech remained relatively clear until the last couple of months; shortly afterward, she started to have difficulty swallowing. In retrospect, this was the beginning of her final decline.

Gen's granddaughter, CA

~ Language remained reasonable until the last six months when Mom struggled seriously to come up with the word she wanted. She was pretty silent the last two months and it was not clear that she understood others the last month.

Helen's daughter, OR

~ Initially, Mom improved after being on the supplements and would carry on conversations. As the disease progressed, she spoke very little.

Helen's daughter, WA

~ Mom had her speech skills; she never lost that. She didn't wear her hearing aid: she said she was afraid she would lose it.

Donna's daughter, IA

~ Mom hung onto basic speech language skills longer than I expected, which was a blessing. After she lost her ability to speak clearly, she showed every indication that she could still understand us until about the last two months. She was also hard of hearing and had refused to wear the hearing aids she was fitted for early in the disease, which didn't help. Lanie's daughter, MN

YOUR THOUGHTS -

_____

_____

_____

_____

_____

_____

_____

_____

_____

_____

_____

_____

_____

_____

The wise man hears one word but understands two. (proverb)

Hygiene challenges

~ Dad was afraid to enter the tub for a shower. It was suggested to put a bright towel in the bottom so they don't think they're stepping into a hole.

Alvin's daughter, IA

~ This was maybe the worst. She would only use 2-3 sheets of toilet tissue and always had feces on hands, clothes, etc. She was difficult to bathe and resisted vigorously.

Mildred's daughter, IA

~ Mom did not like the shower in her assisted living so she mainly cleaned up in the bathroom sink. She did use deodorant but quit using makeup.

Mary's daughter, MN

~ When Mom lost her ability to stand or walk, her hygiene habits were bad. She would wear the same dress for weeks. When she went to the nursing home, the staff said she was "pretty crusty" because of lack of being able to bathe properly.

Matilda's daughter, MN

~ Bathing and clean clothes had become a problem at home. Gerald had difficulty shaving. I had trouble sometimes getting him out for a haircut.

Gerald's wife, IA

~ My Dad is able to clean himself with sponge bathing. He will not accept help from aides who are able to come into the home to assist him with a shower. At this time, we are unsure about how he is doing with the sponge bathing. He doesn't smell, though.

Roy's daughter, MN

~ I am very thankful that hygiene, in general, was never a big issue. In the nursing home, though, I don't think they checked often enough on whether she was brushing her teeth.

Lanie's sister, MN

~ Clarence did take a shower and shaved, washed hair, etc. until about five months before passing. I had to give him the shower, wash hair, etc. then.

Clarence's wife, SC

~ Reatha needed help dressing and going to the bathroom almost from the beginning of her nursing home stay.

Reatha's husband, IA

~ Mom was impeccable with her appearance. Until the day she entered the nursing home, her personal routine stayed the same.

Myra's daughter, MN

~ Carol's hygiene has been very good at this time. She does not shower regularly but does do a sponge bath each morning. She gets her hair cut on a regular basis as she has always kept it quite short.   Carol's husband, MN

~ Bathing became an issue. At first, Mom declined all offers of help, but as time went on, she just went along with suggestions. At the nursing home, she had a weekly hair appointment and I think she looked forward to that because she would tell me about the "old ladies" getting their hair done as well. As time went on, she could no longer brush her own teeth and needed help using the bathroom. When the time for adult diapers arrived – she would have been mortified if she had known she was wearing them – she required assistance going to the bathroom and cleaning up afterward.   Genevieve's daughter, MN

~ When Mom lived at home, she dressed well and looked clean. When I visited, she refused to bathe, claiming she had just taken a bath. I don't really know what was going on but she looked clean. When she moved to an Alzheimer's apartment, they took care of everything.   Mary's stepdaughter, MN

~ I bathe my Mom every other day. I take her to the beauty shop for her hair to be done every week. I still continue to take care of her [hair] coloring as I have for about 20 years.   Charlotte's daughter, TX

~ When Grandma went to the care center, my parents continued to do her laundry and assist with her personal care. My brother and sisters and I assisted as much as we could. I think it helped us still feel connected and affirmed her as our treasure.   Gen's granddaughter, CA

~ After going to the Adult Family Home, Mom fought showers. I think she resented being helped. Her resentment toward being cared for by others endured and only got worse. During this period, she did accept brushing dentures and was self-sufficient with the toilet.   Helen's daughter, OR

~ When we placed her in the Adult Family Home, Mom resisted taking showers or having her hair washed. She resisted the water: it was either too hot or too cold.   Helen's daughter, WA

~ Mom wasn't good about bathing or using deodorant.   Donna's daughter, IA

~ When she lived on her own, Mom did a pretty good job of staying clean although her use of deodorant was not consistent. She did agree to have her hair washed and set once a week; this seemed to help her self-esteem and was a good outing for us. When she went to the nursing home, the steady bathing and hair care schedule was a relief to all of us. Lanie's daughter, MN

YOUR THOUGHTS -

I'm tired of all this business about beauty being only skin-deep.
That's deep enough. What do you want – an adorable pancreas? (Jean Kerr)

Clothing challenges

~ Mom took care of this. She said it was very hard the last night Dad was with her. She cried while sewing nametags in his clothes.
Alvin's daughter, IA

~ Mom didn't like her clothes and only was willing to wear a few items. She considered the others to be hand-me-downs or to have belonged to her mother, even thought Mom had purchased them.
Helen's daughter, WA

~ My sister had to go over and put clothes in the hamper since Mom seemed to forget to change clothes. Every week, we set up a routine and wrote the schedule on the calendar. Very basic but helpful for Mom.
Donna's daughter, IA

~ I knew we were in trouble when, one afternoon, I went to Mom's apartment to pick her up for a doctor's appointment. She was dressed and waiting for me – with her bra worn on the outside of her shirt. Sometimes, she would put on two bras or two shirts. In the nursing home, I resorted to the easy way of getting her dressed – sweatshirt and sweat pants. I sewed little flowers or lace items on the shirts to pretty them up a bit for her. She liked the comfortable feeling and the softness of the fabric. At times, she would be wearing the red shirt with the blue pants or yellow with lavender but she was dressed and clean and that mattered most. I did all of her laundry rather than mix it in with the things at the nursing home. I also labeled each item of clothing and anything else she had. Things had a ways of disappearing anyway.
Genevieve's daughter, MN

~ Clothing is a big issue with my Mom. She is always saying she does not have enough clothes. I just purchased $300 worth of clothes for her and $100 in undergarments. One minute, she likes the clothes and the next she doesn't. She has always had very nice, expensive clothes.
Charlotte's daughter, TX

~ My Mom helped maintain Grandma's wardrobe. She found "simple-to-wear-and-clean" clothes, like sweat suits and embellished them with lace, decorated with ribbon, etc. We made a great fuss over Grandma about how nice she looked. She seemed very contentedly pleased, so we felt better, too.
Gen's granddaughter, CA

~ She always wanted to wear the same thing. We had to start hiding some of these items so that we could get them washed. Then, suddenly, she would hate these favorites and refuse to wear them.
Helen's daughter, OR

~ Dad wore mostly long-sleeved shirts and overalls. Seemed to be cold all of the time. He had no desire to "look good" when we took him out, etc.

Joe's daughter, IA

~ Mother had a few favorite tops that she wore and they always had to have pockets for her tissues. She liked tops and sweaters that were "glitzy" (rhinestones and glitter).

Margaret's daughter, KS

~ Mom complained of her stomach hurting so would wear nothing with a waistband until she was totally out of it. The nursing home wanted sweat suits for warmth and modesty's sake.

Mildred's daughter, IA

~ Mom never seemed to have any problems dressing. When she later moved into the nursing home, she pretty much took care of herself in the dressing area.

Mary's daughter, MN

~ Other than wearing the same dress for a week, the clothing was not a problem. Her strength was bad which kept her from getting clean clothes from closets and drawers.

Matilda's daughter, MN

~ Gerald took off his shoes and socks (just like a two-year-old would). I have seen other patients strip but not Gerald as far I know – just shoes and socks. This became a problem when other patients would take his shoes and we would have to search.

Gerald's wife, IA

~ On occasion, Dad will behave in a bizarre way. He generally is a modest person but some drugs he was put on seemed to magnify his AD. He had himself convinced that he needed an enema and paraded around the house, bottom exposed, wanting one. Sometimes he will have layers of clothes on when it is very warm out. And, sometimes, he forgets to change his clothes and needs to be reminded.

Roy's daughter, MN

~ When I went to her apartment to help her clean, her easy chair [in the living room] was loaded with clothes. I hung them all up and told her to be sure to hang her clothes up as she took them off. The next week, the chair was loaded again. She just kept changing her clothes all the time.

Lanie's sister, MN

~ The last five months, I had to dress him in the morning and help him undress.

Clarence's wife, SC

~ Mom kept her grasp of the progression of clothing (undergarments, then the outer layer) most of the time that she lived by herself but did have a tendency to not dress for the weather (sweatshirts in summer; no coat in winter). In the nursing home, my very modest Mom went through a phase of removing all of her clothes and parading around. Until that phase passed, the staff dressed her in jumpsuits that she couldn't remove.

Lanie's daughter, MN

YOUR THOUGHTS -

_____

_____

_____

_____

_____

_____

_____

_____

_____

_____

_____

_____

_____

_____

Be of good cheer. Do not think of today's failures, but of the success that may come tomorrow. You have set yourself a difficult task, but you will succeed if you persevere; and you will find a joy in overcoming obstacles. (Helen Keller)

_____

_____

_____

_____

_____

_____

_____

_____

_____

_____

_____

_____

_____

_____

_____

Mental challenges

~ My mother did not have hallucinations. She'd forget the daily routine and would always wonder where "Ray" was (my Dad who'd died several years before). Sometimes, I would get up in the morning and she would be in another bedroom because "when those people come home, they don't want me in their bed . . ."   Marie's daughter, MN

~ Dad had his "cats" to take care of. Mom never argued with him about what he "saw".   Alvin's daughter, IA

~ At the very end, we discovered that Dad was full of cancer and he had probably been trying to tell us of what was wrong, but we were unable to understand his complaints enough to follow through with the appropriate steps that would have discovered this earlier. This would have made making him physically more comfortable possible.   Joe's daughter, IA

~ Mom did not hallucinate until she had been in the nursing home for about 18 months and then she would call everyone and tell them that the "kids" (staff) were in the corners laughing at her and stealing from her. My sister was always able to find the things Mom called about.   Matilda's daughter, MN

~ Hallucinations at home were very common – always wanting to know if "those people left" or were they coming back. Common household noises would put him in a panic – things like the refrigerator running or the furnace turning on.   Gerald's wife, IA

~ Dad has been telling stories about people and his past. We are unsure of the truthfulness and have decided that we feel we need to treat them as make-believe. He has become obsessed with watching TV and it seems that some of what he tells us could be things he's seen and then puts family members "into the action".   Roy's daughter, MN

~ After Mother was back living with us, she got up in the middle of the night and began taking pictures, etc. off the walls and putting them on the kitchen table. I never heard her until we came down for breakfast and she said we have to hurry and pack and get ready to go up to Minnesota.   Margaret's daughter, KS

~ Paranoia was the most challenging. She was always sure everyone thought she was "crazy".   Mildred's daughter, IA

~ Lanie's one big problem was with her purse. She "knew" people were coming into her house and she would hide her purse – so well that we had a very hard time finding it.   Lanie's sister, MN

~ Mom's mind played tricks on her many times. She would talk about people who came to visit. It never happened. Things were being "stolen" and later that day, we found them. She said a lady came and borrowed sweaters. Another person came quite regularly to steal her cane. I always managed to find it.   Myra's daughter, MN

~ I just experienced something new. Carol got up and dressed and came down to the living room. She stood in front of the corner knick-knack cabinet and asked me which ones I wanted her to throw out. Obviously, she had a dream about this. I assured her that I would never ask her to throw out anything from this cabinet.   Carol's husband, MN

~ In her apartment, my mother would want to go "upstairs to see my sister, Julia". I would find Mom wandering the halls looking for the way to go upstairs. She called "911" on two different occasions to report that her great-grandchildren who were visiting her were missing – all three of them. When the police called me to come over, Mom insisted the children were gone and she was hysterical. It took a long time to calm her down. The police called my daughter who told them that the three children were at home with her and were just fine. When my Mom talked with my daughter, she became frantic and wouldn't believe the children were all right. She kept saying how sorry she was – that she had just turned her back for a minute and then they were gone. Sometimes, she would go outside and wander the apartment grounds looking for the grandchildren. It was all very sad.   Genevieve's daughter, MN

~ While in Superior, mother thought she saw a man in her car in the garage. She called the police. They knew something was wrong and notified the family. Once, at my home, Mom woke up very upset and unreasonable. For two hours, she tried to explain this experience she had to me. I don't know if it was a bad dream or hallucinations. I don't think it ever happened again, but it was terrible.   Mary's stepdaughter, MN

~ My grandmother had hallucinations and delusions during the final six months of her life. Some of them were honestly very funny and my family is still comforted by those memories. An example: while waiting in hospital admitting, my Grandma told the clerk that her husband would be here but he was golfing. My grandfather died many years earlier and never played golf once in his life.   Gen's granddaughter, CA

~ Mom kept having nightmares that someone was after her. She would yell, "Leave me alone, get out of here, you are hurting me!"   Helen's daughter, WA

~ One of the hardest things for us to work through was Mom's hallucinations. They were worst when she was still in her house – she was sure there were people living in the closet under the stairs in the basement. I smile as I type this because it sounds like a sleazy movie title but, at the time, there was nothing funny about it. She did not get past this phase until we moved her to her apartment - on the 11th floor of the building. Soon after the move, she said that someone was looking in the window but when I pointed out that that would be impossible because of the height, she never brought "them" up again. The worst of her hallucinations was the one that got her evicted from her apartment. She was thoroughly frightened and sure that someone had hit her in the stomach as she wandered around the main floor of her apartment building in the middle of the night. The saddest part for me was when she attempted to write out what happened to her for me because she saw that I didn't understand her. The writing was just gibberish – various letters together, no words. It breaks my heart to imagine the frustration she was experiencing.

Lanie's daughter, MN

YOUR THOUGHTS -

_____

_____

_____

_____

_____

_____

_____

_____

_____

> **Our memories are card indexes, consulted and then put back in disorder by authorities whom we do not control.** (Cyril Connolly, *The Unquiet*)

Rare "in the moment" times to cherish

~ I knew my Grandma's health was failing. I was scheduled to return to California and had to go. She looked at me as I was leaving and said, "Thank you for everything you've ever done for me. I've always loved you." I cried then as I cry now as I write this. She died 2 or 3 days later.   Gen's granddaughter, CA

~ When we would walk down the hall at the nursing home, Mother would introduce me to everyone, even though I had met everyone before.   Margaret's daughter, KS

~ She responded to my singing old hymns and would either sing with me or would be very quiet to listen. Mildred's daughter, IA

~ So far, Dad has the ability to respond to those talking with him. On occasion, he may not know someone or a pet. So far, he has stayed pretty positive through the disease.   Roy's daughter, MN

~ Carol still communicates well with everyone although not for great lengths of time. Crowd noises bother her a lot so we do not go to concerts or sporting events any more.   Carol's husband, MN

~ In November, just before Thanksgiving, I went to the nursing home to see my Mom. Coffee and cookies were available so we walked to the cafeteria. As we were sitting with our coffee, she began to talk to me in a very clear manner. She asked me questions about family members, talked about the weather, made small talk, and even knew what time it was and that it was close to Thanksgiving. I remember saying, "We'll have to shop for Christmas cards soon." It was as if a window opened in her brain and all was right with the world again. Wow! We had a great visit, and I went home to tell my husband that I thought she was back to her normal self and we could bring her to our home to live. I was elated! The next morning, my "real" Mom was gone again – replaced with the woman captured by this damn disease that took her heart and soul from us. I thank God for that one glorious day I was able to spend with her.   Genevieve's daughter, MN

~ Mom communicated best when we talked about her growing up. She had lots of stories. The more recent the years we asked about, the less she remembered.   Donna's daughter, IA

~ We cherished her smile when she was in a good mood because you never knew when she would get mad. Helen's daughter, OR

~ Until close to the end, Mom always responded to people who talked to her directly, one-on-one. However, once she started to lose her ability to really verbally communicate, I don't remember any extended length of time when she could converse more than two or three sentences. I recall one time at the nursing home when I was sitting on the floor next to her during a program that was being presented and Mom started to stroke my head. It felt so wonderful to have this spontaneous display of affection – I hardly dared breathe for fear she'd stop. The AD caregiver's soul yearns for moments like that.

Lanie's daughter, MN

When everything else seems to diminish, the appreciation of beauty is on the increase.

(Bernard Berenson, *Sunset and Twilight*)

YOUR THOUGHTS -

_____

_____

_____

_____

_____

_____

_____

_____

_____

_____

_____

Recalling the not-so-distant past and other interesting thought patterns

~ Mom began calling Dad "Papa" after she entered the nursing home. This was what she had always called her father. She began calling me "Mama". She avoided having to call anyone by name. She continued to call Dad "Papa" until he died.

Mildred's daughter, IA

~ My Dad was in the nursing home [first]. When my sister and I came back to the house after getting Dad settled, Mom had removed from sight everything of my Dad's. After he passed away, it was like he never existed. Mom often commented that her home was the home that she had with her parents. This made me feel very hurt as I couldn't understand why she never felt she and Dad had created a home for us.

Matilda's daughter, MN

~ Gerald was always looking for or worried about his mother. One time, still at home, in late afternoon, he said we had to go milk the cows. I said I had never milked a cow and never lived on a farm. He said, "Well, you'd better learn now – the cows need to be milked!"

Gerald's wife, IA

~ Over the years, Dad is very convinced of "how to eat" and of trying all sorts of supplements. Then he presses his opinions onto others. He has spent many dollars over the years trying this supplement and then that one. I have seen him become adamant with his views on nutrition and is obsessed with vitamins/supplements. It is hard to see him try to fix himself in this way because the vitamin companies are taking his money and haven't seen much improvement. And, after all he says, he does not practice and he eats whatever and forgets to take the vitamins.

Roy's daughter, MN

~ When I would talk about our Mom, Lanie would look me in the eye and say, "I hated her." Lanie was a middle child and always felt neglected. If she was [neglected], it wasn't obvious at the time. We didn't talk about the past much because she couldn't remember it most of the time.

Lanie's sister, MN

~ Clarence's mother passed away in March, 1985. In June, 2003, he wanted to take a trip and go see his mother in Pennsylvania. He said he did not know she had died.

Clarence's wife, SC

~ My grandmother, in her final six months or so, frequently "talked" to deceased family and friends as if they were in the room with her. As a nurse, I have seen this in patients nearing death. It was unnerving to see this in my now-confused Grandma.

Gen's granddaughter, CA

~ In the nursing home, Mom asked several times during the last four months, "Do I still have my little green house?" It really tore at my heart because we sold it to pay for her care. So I'd answer, "Mom, it's still there." She was satisfied. The home had bingo twice a week and a music entertainment one afternoon. Until the last month, Mom went to everything just to help stimulate her mind. The sing-alongs were nice, especially the German songs. At first, she sang some and later, just tapped her finger.   Myra's daughter, MN

~ It surprised me that my mother spoke more about her two sisters and her brother than she did my father. An interesting thought pattern was that even though Mom forgot my name and who I was (sometimes I became her sister, Frances), she never ever forgot my husband and never faltered with his name. She was quite clear who he was right up to the end. I will admit that hurt a bit – just a little sting.   Genevieve's daughter, MN

~ Once, while having dinner at my house, Mom stated, "I wish someone would take me to see my sister." The next week, we took her to Superior to see her sister (her sister also had Alzheimer's). The sisters stared at each other and both said, "That's not my sister."   Mary's stepdaughter, MN

~ Mother calls me other names at times. She can never remember our Jack Russell mix dog's name. Charlotte's daughter, TX

~ Mom asked about her parents as if she were a little girl.   Helen's daughter, OR

~ When Mom was put in the Adult Family Home, she would ask, "When are my parents going to come get me?" She would forget who I was and associate me with her older sister.   Helen's daughter, WA

~ For some time, we looked at a lot of old pictures she had taken and she could talk about who they were. Then one day, she showed no interest. She kept looking for Ray (my Dad) to come home and wondered where he was. This was every day.   Marie's daughter, MN

~ Dad would pull out furniture and "work" on it like it was a piece of machinery he had worked on in years past. Sometimes, you just had to laugh at the things he did.   Alvin's daughter, IA

~ Early on, Alvin brought up visiting his mother who had died many years past. Then he realized she was gone. He also knew something was wrong when his brother-in-law died when he didn't come see him.   Alvin's wife, IA

~ Mom had always mixed up my aunt and me. This continued and we no longer corrected her. She and my father were divorced in 1970 and she did not talk about him with me much in the interim (although was fine it if I brought him up in conversation). She began to look for him to come and see her in the nursing home and became more obsessed with him and their past life, often breaking into sobs. At this point, the nursing home staff recommended that we take her off of the Aricept as it was working just enough to let her remember things that would upset her. That decision took me a few days to work through emotionally because it meant that there was no more help medically available to her. I needed to accept that the decline that Aricept had slowed was now going to accelerate.

Lanie's daughter, MN

YOUR THOUGHTS -

_____

_____

_____

_____

_____

_____

_____

_____

_____

_____

_____

Where are the songs of spring? Ay, where are they?
Think not of them - thou hast thy music too. (Keats)

_____

_____

_____

_____

_____

_____

_____

_____

_____

_____

_____

_____

_____

_____

_____

Signs of frustrations in the patient; acting out

~ In the nursing home, Mom could be very angry and physical. Although she was small, it was nothing for her to swat someone if she didn't like what they did or said. It didn't matter if it was another patient or an aide. When we were there, Mom would completely ignore other patients. She was very upset if they sat with us or we talked to any of them.

Mary's daughter, MN

~ Mom was almost never angry at the nursing home staff, but was quite often (very often) angry at my sister and me for putting her in the nursing home. Once in a while, she would become angry at a staff person if they tried to get her to do something she didn't want to do but nothing was physical. She just wouldn't talk to them for a while. Matilda's daughter, MN

~ Gerald was generally complacent, willing to cooperate and do what the aide wanted. But once he did throw the aide against the wall when he was trying to give Gerald a shower. Another time, Gerald knocked an aide's tooth out when they were trying to get Gerald to sit on the toilet.

Gerald's wife, IA

~ My Mother, if suffering, suffered in silence. She would grumble once in a while when she couldn't find something or do something. She did get angry at me when I did housework. She thought I was someone else and she would yell at me, "Mary Ann does the housework – who are you? You're not supposed to vacuum. Mary Ann does the vacuuming." Of course, it was me all the time.

Marie's daughter, MN

~ Dad "flunked out" of one nursing home and was labeled "dangerous" which made finding another one difficult. He wanted help from the staff and could not make them understand him which ended with him threatening a staff member with a chair. In retrospect, I feel he was in a great deal of pain and wanted relief from it – possibly thinking they were denying him painkillers when the fact was that they did not know of his pain. I had to run to Lake City to the nursing home several nights to get Dad cleaned up or to bed when he got to where he would not let them do any personal things for him.

Joe's daughter, IA

~ Mother was not pleased to have someone help her with her bath. She didn't want anyone to see her naked.

Margaret's daughter, KS

~ Mom was frustrated at home already. She was cooperative with me and the staff. At first, she did have a problem sharing a room.

Myra's daughter, MN

~ Dad at times becomes angry. I think the realities of AD hit him and he becomes fearful of what is taking place within that he cannot control. I have discussed these situations with others within the family. Dad was a violent drunk when he was intoxicated. Studies show that anger outbursts can be a part of a person who has AD and we are prepared to deal with it but – it won't be easy, though.
Roy's daughter, MN

~ My mother was a very, very prejudiced person and would have never allowed an African-American nurse to care for her under normal circumstances. One of the aides [at the nursing home] was black and she became one of my Mom's favorites. There was an absence of anger toward the end, and the only real frustration (early on) was when she couldn't find her purse or couldn't remember a certain word.
Genevieve's daughter, MN

~ Clarence would get really frustrated if I would try to help him remember something or correct whatever he was saying.
Clarence's wife, SC

~ Mother would get angry when she thought we wanted her out of her house. She was much sweeter once we moved her to St. Paul [to be by her children].
Mary's stepdaughter, MN

~ My Mom has very few episodes of pure anger. She will scream and shout once in a while when she feels she cannot get her way (right away).
Charlotte's daughter, TX

~ Mom would swing her cane at caregivers and yell and push the caregiver away when being given a shower. She refused to have her hair washed and, after she was incontinent, she fought being cleaned up. She pushed food away and said it was crap. Mom was angry a lot.
Helen's daughter, OR

~ Mom would threaten her caregiver by waving her cane Once, she hit a caregiver.
Helen's daughter, WA

~ Mom never was physically uncooperative with my aunt or me, but did show frustration and anger to the nursing home staff. She'd pull hair or take a swing at the aides if they wanted her to do something she didn't want to do. She was also often adamant about not wanting to share a table in the dining room with certain other residents of the AD unit. Fortunately, she always calmed down.

Lanie's daughter, MN

YOUR THOUGHTS -

_____

_____

_____

_____

_____

_____

_____

_____

_____

_____

_____

_____

_____

How you, the caregiver, handle(d) your frustrations and anger

~ In the beginning, I was very angry, very frustrated and felt cheated out of the "golden years". I was angry at God and jealous of those couples enjoying life. Again, support groups show others are thinking those thoughts, too, and I was not alone. We could express those thoughts and it was alright.   Gerald's wife, IA

~ The only time I ever got angry at Mom was the time of the nose[bleed] problems when she kept pulling out the packing. It was a total frustration for me. I regret getting angry to this day.   Milta's son, KS

~ I was sad, because I knew what was coming after my mother-in-law died, but grateful that my husband was here to give me strength.   Margaret's daughter, KS

~ I felt a lot of guilt for living 400 miles away when she needed me. I felt I could have done so much to keep her home if I had been closer. I stayed with her several days while Dad had surgery and I nearly went crazy myself. Mildred's daughter, IA

~ Going to see Mom was very stressful for me. I would return home from my visits all stressed out and found I had to lay down for a 10 minute nap. Being an only child, everything fell on me.   Mary's daughter, MN

~ We just listened to Mom when she was angry or frustrated and would say, "I feel bad that you are feeling <sad or angry or frustrated>", which would usually defuse Mom's problem at the time.   Matilda's daughter, MN

~ The thing for myself through this experience of being the major caregiver for my Dad is that I now have to make decisions for him, who can't. My Dad is now reverting to childhood and if he lives long enough, he will become silent. It saddens me greatly and I grieve through the stages of this disease as I watch my Dad deteriorate and I cannot do a thing except assist him through this. Although I have siblings to assist me, I still find myself giving the majority of the care. God sustains me with an ever-flowing supply of his grace and a husband who gives of himself to assist, too. And a loving daughter who wants to help Grandpa!   Roy's daughter, MN

~ There is no real way to deal with the frustration of Alzheimer's. It is always there and you learn to live with it – never accept it. The anger, also, never goes away.   Lanie's sister, MN

~ I was really upset as the disease progressed. He entered the VA hospital in August, 2003. The first week in September, I had him home for seven days but he had to go back. Every day [while at home] he fell once or twice and I had to get friends to come in and get him up.

Clarence's wife, SC

~ I was mad as hell and so guilt-ridden that I could barely function some days. How could this happen to this woman who had been so strong and in-charge? Could I have seen this coming sooner? Should I have done more interventions and then this would not have gotten out of control? <u>I want to be in control</u> – and this was something out of my hands entirely. I had no siblings, and even though I had a large and caring support system, the ultimate decisions were mine alone. How could I make these kinds of decisions when I was so exhausted and my mind felt like it was full of soft pudding? I could not do this – I had no strength left to even get through the day, let alone make life-and-death decisions for my Mom. I would lie awake at night with thoughts bouncing around in my head so much that I could not complete one sentence in my thoughts without another starting to take its place. I felt like I was the one that was losing her mind. My God, was AD contagious? In the dark of night, I was sure it was and I knew I had not been vaccinated against it!! God help ME for once – I can't cope any longer.

Genevieve's daughter, MN

~ In the early stages, it was frustrating. When she lost things, she wouldn't let you help her. Later, it was so sad when she did things that would have embarrassed her: poor conversation, bad table manners, etc.

Mary's stepdaughter, MN

~ I get frustrated at times. Mom will nag me constantly at times until I have to go to my room and tell her I must have some "down time". She is unaware of the nagging and says she doesn't nag.

Charlotte's daughter, TX

~ The day we left Grandma at the care facility, I cried for hours. I still wonder if this was the right decision but I believe it was. I hated living so far from my family. I had responsibilities in California but wanted to be in Minnesota with my family.

Gen's granddaughter, CA

~ I was frustrated that Mom's problems consumed my family's life. I had trouble sleeping and developed high blood pressure. The situation was overwhelming.

Helen's daughter, WA

~ In the beginning, I was angry at the diagnosis and at myself for not getting her to the doctor for the diagnosis sooner. As the disease progressed, I was just so sad. The highway exit to the nursing home was on my way home from work and there were days that I just could not stop and see her. I journaled a lot to try and work through my feelings and anger at the other things I had to deal with regarding her care. Ridiculously, I HATED that I was an only child more than anything – it was all on me. There were some days where it was real easy to fall into the self-pity trap.   Lanie's daughter, MN

YOUR THOUGHTS -

_____

_____

_____

_____

_____

_____

_____

_____

_____

_____

_____

_____

_____

When you give vent to your feelings, anger leaves you. (proverb)

Housing decisions; dealing with possessions

~ In the beginning, we tried to get Mom interested in buying a house in an assisted living community. She would have no part. We tried an apartment with assisted living. Mom was very angry. We eventually talked her into Adult Family Home care many months later which she eventually settled into pretty well, but she was still a difficult resident. We eventually moved her back home with in-home caregivers (1.5 years) which went reasonably well for about one year, after which Mom did not even recognize that she was in her own home. She kept saying she wanted to go home. Most of her possessions are still in the house as we await final probate/estate settlement.   Helen's daughter, OR

~ We moved Mom to an Alzheimer's apartment. Her bed, dresser, couch, TV, etc. went with her and that made the transition much better. The house was sold and possessions divided among the children. She had no financial problems.
                                                                        Mary's stepdaughter, MN

~ Mother lives with me and continues to do so. I have had her for about seven years. Mother sees her doctor on a regular basis. She cannot take certain meds due to the side effects. Fortunately, the AD is moving slowly. I handle all of Mom's needs – spiritual, financial and health. She is unable to take care of herself, period.   Charlotte's daughter, TX

~ I held on to Mom's apartment for three months, thinking she could come back. That meant three months' rent paid for an empty apartment. Luckily, my Mom was able to cover her nursing home expenses with her monthly checks and her savings. After she died, there was very little money left that she and my dad had worked so hard to save and invest. It's Hell to get old! When I finally was able to let the apartment go, I called each of my five children and told them to meet me at 10:00 a.m. one Saturday morning and to bring their trucks and empty boxes. I had already taken the things that meant something special to me, so when my children arrived, I left the apartment and told them to divide up their grandmother's possessions among themselves. Never before had I been so damn proud of my kids. They divided things and never argued as they accomplished this very sad task, and they did it all with caring and grace   Genevieve's daughter, MN

~ We sold Mom's home to finance her care. That's all she had with a small Social Security check. We furnished her room with things from her bedroom – a lamp, mirror tray, kissing angels (Myra and Fritz), pictures off of her walls from home, a chair she always sat in, etc.   Myra's daughter, MN

~ At this point, we live in a two-level townhome and we are doing just fine with the steps at this time although I believe this will be a concern in the future.

Carol's husband, MN

~ I took her clothes over [to the nursing home] on Sunday and Reatha on Monday. When I walked out the door of the nursing home and heard the door click shut and I knew I had just locked my wife in, it really hit me just what was taking place. Reatha was very different than any of the other residents there. She would pace the hallway and upset chairs along the way. She didn't hurt anyone but was always on the move. She didn't sleep in her bed for the first two years she was there. She always slept in a recliner in the activity room. Reatha would hardly stop walking long enough to eat; many times they had to try and feed her on the move. The director of the unit pretty much took Reatha under her wing and took care of her. The state wouldn't allow restraints to be used.

Reatha's husband, IA

~ When Mom was unable to walk, she decided she would try the nursing home. She convinced herself that she would be in the nursing home a month and then be able to go home. They tried therapy but she never got out of the wheelchair again to do much walking. She was able to be in the assisted living unit but only for a short while until she fell. The staff needed her closer to them. We were able to have her in a private room except for the first month in the home. Too bad that people going into a nursing home can't all have a private room. Mom had nursing home insurance [long-term care insurance], which was most helpful. We never needed public assistance.

Matilda's daughter, MN

~ The transition to the nursing home was fairly easy. My friend, Mr. D, and I had visited nursing homes so I knew where I wanted Gerald to be. One morning, Mr. D and another friend, a retired nurse, came over for coffee. Mr. D. said we would go for a drive. At the nursing home, we said we wanted to visit someone. Gerald immediately joined a group of patients sitting in a circle playing catch – just as they did at day care.

Gerald's wife, IA

~ Dad doesn't have many possessions and is still able to live in his home. We take one day at a time. We have gone through my parents' finances and have aided them to simplify their expenses and to evaluate what they have in Social Security, pensions, etc. We are prepared to aid them with state and insurance paperwork, etc. to help them to get the care they need as the need arises. Their wish is to die in their home and we would like them to be able to live that desire out, but we are realistic, too, and understand that they may need to be placed in a nursing home when the care needed is beyond what I can give.

Roy's daughter, MN

131

~ After Mom was no longer able to work to pay off her debts, I got her on a list for public housing where you pay according to your ability. When she got her TINY apartment, we moved what she needed and had a sale for the rest of her possessions. After the wandering episode at the public housing apartment building prompted an eviction notice, I had to find her a nursing home <u>fast</u>. I was so blessed to find one that had an AD unit just for women. I had already done a ton of paperwork to get her into the apartment so was prepared with the information to get her into the nursing home quickly. As a result of losing everything to her gambling, Mom needed public assistance to pay the remainder of the cost of the nursing home after her pension and Social Security checks were applied to the fees.   Lanie's daughter, MN

YOUR THOUGHTS -

_____

_____

_____

_____

_____

_____

_____

_____

_____

_____

_____

You gain strength, courage, and confidence by every experience in which you really stop to look fear in the face. You must do the thing which you think you cannot do. (Eleanor Roosevelt)

_____

_____

_____

_____

_____

_____

_____

_____

_____

_____

_____

_____

_____

_____

_____

Medical decisions at this point

~ In the beginning, we tried supplements, herbals and vitamins. We also tried various antidepressants but they all seemed to either upset Mom's stomach or have ill- or no effects. Eventually, her nighttime hallucinations led us to sleeping aids and other anti-hallucinogenic drugs. Each of these had either limited or short-lived effects.   Helen's daughter, OR

~ When I would go over and visit her, we would walk several miles in the hallway, 25 rounds = 1 mile, then I would put her in her room and sit in the doorway so she couldn't get out. It was a very hard several months. Dr. L. finally decided to try a medication that he was using for another disease. It really worked and didn't sedate her. She still walked but not with the determination that she did before.   Reatha's husband, IA

~ Upon entering the home, Mom's cane was replaced with a walker. For several years, now, her left hip was giving her pain. Meds didn't seem to help much. Finally, she went into a wheelchair. Mom had several seizures. Instead of having a battery of tests, MRI, etc., the doctor felt they could be controlled with meds. If the problem was a tumor, they wouldn't recommend surgery anyway. Just before entering the home, Mom had a dental check and eye exams. Myra's daughter, MN

~ I make all of Carol's medical appointments and go with her when seeing doctors. Staying in tune with what is real and imagined sometimes can be difficult. Thankfully, her doctor is very understanding and loving in her care for Carol.
           Carol's husband, MN

~ Mother was examined by a physician's assistant often while at the home. At one point, they took her off Cognex, stating that it no longer helped. Two weeks later, they resumed the Cognex as the nurses felt she was less alert without it.
           Mary's stepdaughter, MN

~ Mother refuses to even discuss a nursing home. I will have her until she is gone or I am gone – one or the other.
           Charlotte's daughter, TX

~ Gerald was mobile, still walking. He was continent most of the time. The nursing home practically insisted on my signing a DNR [Do Not Resuscitate]. I refused at first, but my doctor convinced me to sign. Each step is an acknowledgement of the decline.   Gerald's wife, IA

~ In the last year, my Dad has been through six surgeries. It has been hard to deal with because he is not only mentally deteriorating, but physically, too! When the prospect of another surgery is mentioned, I cringe and pray for wisdom. When does someone say enough is enough???
Roy's daughter, MN

~ After entering the hospital in August, Clarence would sit in a wheelchair and visit with others there. Then in September, he was not out of bed for anything. [I also made the decision about] no feeding tube or anything to keep him alive. That was a hard decision for me and my daughter. We could see he was really going downhill and they did not recommend it, either.
Clarence's wife, SC

~ When Mother entered the nursing home, they were concerned that she might fall as she walked with her knees bent. She was a skier in her youth and said that bending her knees gave her better balance. She was known at the home as "Maggie".
Margaret's daughter, KS

~ About March, 1991, I ran quickly to the store. There was snow and my Mother had fallen on the back porch and broken her hip. Three weeks later she died after being in a nursing home for three days after her hip surgery.
Marie's daughter, MN

~ Dad was walking slowly by this time. He eventually fell and broke his hip and then was placed in a special "Merry Walker" that allowed him to walk but also sit when he tired.
Alvin's daughter, IA

~ Dad made DNR decision many years ago. He had signed papers and had given Power of Attorney for health care to my brother.
Joe's daughter, IA

~ Mom was given no meds after the move [to the smaller facility]. My Dad and Mom shared a room the last two years of his life.
Mildred's daughter, IA

~ When Mom entered the nursing home, she was unable to walk, see or hear very well. She had used a walker while still at home. She refused hearing aids because no one was ever able to hear that had them.
Matilda's daughter, MN

~ I had to get two doctors to certify Mom's condition to activate the Durable Power of Attorney. I would consult with my sister but, ultimately, all decisions were made by me.
Helen's daughter, WA

~ When Mom entered the nursing home, she was evaluated for mobility, which resulted in her getting a walker. This really helped her as she had scoliosis that had given her back pain for years. I made the decision for "DNR" (Do Not Resuscitate) and no feeding tube when and if she could no longer eat. Mom was very healthy physically and there was no reason to think that she would not be with us for a number of years, if she didn't break a hip or get pneumonia. But then, what did I know?
Lanie's daughter, MN

YOUR THOUGHTS -

_____

_____

_____

_____

_____

_____

_____

_____

_____

_____

_____

_____

More money decisions

~ Mom handled her own money until she could no longer see to write checks. My sister always saw to it Mom had a little money in her wallet until she started giving it away and would then call my sister for more. My sister finally told everyone that she would pay the beauty operator once a month. Mom always complained that she never had any money because her daughters had spent it all.
Matilda's daughter, MN

~ We did have nursing home insurance [long-term care insurance] – just for $50 per day for four years. The cost was $100 a day for a two-bed room. So the insurance helped enough that I could privately pay. Medications and haircuts were extra. Of course, I kind of resented our hard-earned savings going to the nursing home, but was also very glad I could pay and proud I did.
Gerald's wife, IA

~ So far, Dad has the ability to hold some money and spend it. The issue for me is deciding when I need to step in because so many things for Dad have been taken away, and he feels that his independence is going away with them. As a family, we are trying to oversee the finances and have an awareness that we may need to step in sooner than planned before anything gets out of hand with finances.
Roy's daughter, MN

~ There was a long period of time when my niece went through hell (excuse the word) because of Lanie's financial situation. We both were aware of Lanie's gambling but not of the way she was getting money to support her habit. Lanie's sister, MN

~ Before my Mother was diagnosed, we went to an attorney and drew up a will and a living will. Because I took care of her at home – cooking, washing clothes and keeping her clean – there were no huge expenses. [Later], she didn't know me, but knew I was someone she could trust.
Marie's daughter, MN

~ When Mom entered the home, we sold her little green house. This is a very difficult thing to do. We did buy a beautiful lounge chair for Mom to have in the family area. After she passed, we left the chair and Mom's clothes for others to use.
Myra's daughter, MN

~ I have taken over all decisions regarding our finances including where Carol's IRAs and 401Ks are deposited.
Carol's husband, MN

~ I had been taking care of Mom's finances for years, so it was up to me to make all the arrangements. My husband was a huge help with all of the paperwork – bless his heart! My Mom was content knowing she had a few dollars in her bedside cosmetic-bag "purse".

Genevieve's daughter, MN

~ Mother lost a lot of money in a bad contractor transaction. This was probably the very beginning of her AD. She refused to listen to me and lost about $50,000. Dad was too sick to step in. She would not have listened to him, either.

Charlotte's daughter, TX

~ Early on, Mom agreed to my sister having Power of Attorney and Mom was happy to be relieved of financial burdens. There were no money disasters. Mom did report to Adult Family Home caregivers that we put her there so that we could take her money. That hurt, even though it was not true.

Helen's daughter, OR

~ Mom was always a good money manager. We did some changes in her investments to help with her tax liability. She thought we didn't think she knew what she was doing. We had to keep reassuring her that she had done so well it was costing her more in taxes.

Donna's daughter, IA

~ Thankfully, my parents had the foresight to take care of this issue before it was necessary. This is something I would recommend for anyone with aging parents. The time of crisis is NOT the time to be dealing with this issue.

Gen's granddaughter, CA

~ Because Mom had gotten into such financial difficulties, she ended up with no assets. Once the paperwork was completed for her to receive assistance from the county to pay the nursing home fees, every penny was accounted for. She was allowed to put $69 per month into a special account for clothes, getting her hair done, etc. The rest of her pension and Social Security went toward paying for her stay at the nursing home. Fortunately, her needs were small so this turned out to be OK.   Lanie's daughter, MN

YOUR THOUGHTS -

_____

_____

_____

_____

_____

_____

_____

_____

_____

_____

_____

_____

Troubles no one wants to steal; good deeds, no one can. (proverb)

The patient's faith-based habits

~ Mom was a very regular churchgoer but quit going while she was still home because "they thought she was crazy". Not responsive to pastoral visits.   Mildred's daughter, IA

~ Mom did attend church services at the home. Unfortunately, she mainly slept through them.   Mary's daughter, MN

~ My parents always went to church. Once Mom figured out she wasn't ever going to be able to return to her house, her faith was never acknowledged very much. She never refused a minister's visit but never talked about his visits either.
                                                                                            Matilda's daughter, MN

~ The nursing home was Lutheran (we are United Church of Christ). They would take Gerald to services but he would take off his shoes and socks and wander off. So they had to discontinue taking him.   Gerald's wife, IA

~ Dad was raised Catholic and is very set in his beliefs. When I talk with him about his beliefs, I ask him, "What are you going to say to Jesus when you see Him?" Sadly, Dad tells me to have my own religion and he will have his. He no longer attends church or desires to do so.   Roy's daughter, MN

~ My sister was a very Christian woman but had not been associated with a church for years. Just before Lanie became ill, we were going to different churches to find one we both liked so we could belong to one again.   Lanie's sister, MN

~ The last of the seven years, she did not go to church. Up until then, she went with me. She would go up to Communion and take the host – I would guide her back to the pew. I think she knew this was something very significant. Marie's daughter, MN

~ Dad was a faithful Lutheran. Even to the end, he would say the Lord's Prayer completely. When startled, he quieted down when hymns were sung.   Alvin's daughter, IA

~ Mom had a church membership but once she lost her car, she didn't want to go. She had kind of stopped going long before that because she couldn't hear.   Donna's daughter, IA

~ We took Mother to church along with another lady who was in her 90's. It was good for Mother to have someone nearer her age to talk to. We started picking up Anita when my mother-in-law was living with us.   Margaret's daughter, KS

~ We were members of a Methodist church and Clarence went up until he entered the hospital.   Clarence's wife, SC

~ Faith was always a big part in Mom's life. She went to church faithfully every Sunday with Gene and me. Her last year at home, she decided to stay at home. She said her prayers and waited every Sunday for me to bring her Holy Communion. This she appreciated very much.   Myra's daughter, MN

~ Carol still attends services on a regular basis. We attend a couples' Bible study with three other couples once a month. She still says that she enjoys them but just listens (although she never did participate much before). Carol's husband, MN

~ My mother was a "cradle Catholic" and while she could still think clearly, she never lost her faith in God. However, there was a priest at her parish she absolutely did not like or respect. I never requested that he visit her in the nursing home. Mass was offered once a week at the facility, as was the Rosary. We attended these as long as she was able. The very last time we went to Mass, Mom was having a horrible day – she was jittery and could not seem to sit still. Finally, about halfway through, she stood up and said, "Let's get the hell out of here!" And this from a woman who would never, ever swear – and especially not during Mass. The incident still makes me giggle.   Genevieve's daughter, MN

~ With no car, Mom was unable to get to Mass. After she moved here, we took turns taking her to Sunday Mass. Eventually, her behavior at church was inappropriate (not knowing what to do with the Communion host, playing with babies, etc.), so we stopped taking her.   Mary's stepdaughter, MN

~ My Mom is a true believer and has continued with her faith. We are in the process of finding a church she feels comfortable in. She likes the Presbyterian church we visited recently – we may join that one. On some Sundays, I have a hard time getting her going to attend church. I feel if she could find one she liked, she would get up in time to go.   Charlotte's daughter, TX

~ Mom had been Catholic but had not been to church in years. She would have nothing to do with discussions about God. She would say "why me", which I interpreted to mean, "why did God do this to me (or let this happen to me)?"
                                                Helen's daughter, OR

~ Mom was a Lutheran but had not been a regular churchgoer since her divorce from my father. The nursing home was affiliated with a faith so there were regular visits by a minister and a priest who led services with prayers and singing. Mom enjoyed these, but I have no idea if she grasped the significance.   Lanie's daughter, MN

YOUR THOUGHTS -

Nothing is permanent but change. (Heraclitus (quoted by Diogenes))

Care conferences and decisions

~ My sister attended the care conferences and the staff were always praising Mom as to how well she was doing and that she was always pleasant. We were convinced they were talking about someone else.   Matilda's daughter, MN

~ My sister-in-law attended these due to Dad's hearing loss. She would then relay all the information to the rest of us.   Mildred's daughter, IA

~ Mother entered the nursing home very angry. At our first conference, it was stated by the staff that she was bitter and very upset. Later, we were told that she finally accepted her life there and became a favorite.   Mary's daughter, MN

~ Trips to the doctor can be a few trips a week. Otherwise, we settle in and go every other week. Sometimes, home care will come in but Dad sends them away. I am the one who he will accept care from. When a nurse comes, Dad will allow himself to be checked over.   Roy's daughter, MN

~ My sister, Joan, and I attended the care conferences together. Each time, another health problem was explained to us. The disease was winning. Finally, Mom was place on oxygen which she kept for two months.   Myra's daughter, MN

~ Carol's last evaluation was that there seemed to be very little progression in the disease. We see her regular doctor every three months just to keep her in touch with Carol. Carol enjoys these visits because of the loving nature of her doctor.   Carol's husband, MN

~ Same old, same old. Pretty much the staff said, "Yes, she's here – she's doing as well as can be expected." Well, it's not what I wanted to hear. I wanted to be told she was going to be her old self again – a woman who could match her clothes, keep track of her belongings and take care of her finances. It was not to be.   Genevieve's daughter, MN

~ We had care conferences twice yearly. Mom's decline was very gradual, over several years (less language, less alert, etc.)   Mary's stepdaughter, MN

~ My sister had to drive almost every aspect of Mom's care. Only after the visiting nurse was ordered by the doctor, did anyone take much interest in Mom. They did offer options and make recommendations to the doctor. Their efforts helped us get some of the drugs that temporarily helped Mom's hallucinations.   Helen's daughter, OR

~ The nursing home had regularly scheduled care conferences to which the family was invited. My aunt and I always attended. A dietician, the head nurse, the social worker, etc. reviewed Mom's condition with us. There was never any good news – the best we could hope for was that she was stable. The ultimate care conference was one-on-one with the head nurse telling me that it was time to bring in hospice.   Lanie's daughter, MN

If you find it in your heart to care for somebody else, you will have succeeded. (Maya Angelou)

YOUR THOUGHTS -

Grief counseling

~ In our case, members of the family used each other as sounding boards. Sometimes, you just have to understand God gives only what we can bear. We have been given a full measure of heartache besides Mom's disease. Myra's daughter, MN

~ I've always been a positive-type person: even as a recovering alcoholic, I don't get down on myself. The men's group and my part-time job helps a lot if there is sadness setting in. Carol's husband, MN

~ My friends and family became my greatest support network. Their understanding of my family needs was a great comfort (especially work colleagues). Gen's granddaughter, CA

~ I grieved over the loss of my mother long before she died. Piece by piece, she died in front of me. By the time she stopped breathing, I was ready. Helen's daughter, OR

~ We all shared with each other and my brother-in-law who was trained in counseling. Donna's daughter, IA

~ No counseling. I continued to work part-time as the dedicated volunteers came on Tuesday, Wednesday and Thursday afternoons. I became grumpy at work – lots of things bothered me. Marie's daughter, MN

~ I talked with my pastor once around Christmas her first year in the nursing home when I was really grieving and he was helpful as his father had AD. Mildred's daughter, IA

~ Mother blamed me for everything, especially putting her in a home. She would get very angry with me. I felt very guilty in putting Mother "away". Mary's daughter, MN

~ I counted on the support group I had joined. My husband was a very good listener. Matilda's daughter, MN

~ The support groups were my counseling – still are and I continue going so as to help newcomers to this disease and to support others as deaths come. Gerald's wife, IA

~ I pray often and God answers prayers! Family and friends have been very supportive with a listening ear and words of wisdom. Through the church I attend, there are quite a few that have walked the road of caring for a parent. They truly can sympathize. Roy's daughter, MN

~ I did not use any of the formal grief counseling services that were available. At the time, I felt that taking time to go to the sessions that were offered seemed like "just one more thing" to deal with. Looking back, that seems pretty shortsighted. I did journal which helped me work through the bad times. I also could vent with my friends and family. To their credit, they never rolled their eyes at the thought of hearing about Mom yet again.   Lanie's daughter, MN

How small and selfish is sorrow. But it bangs one about until one is senseless.
(Elizabeth, Queen Mother of England)

YOUR THOUGHTS -

_____

_____

_____

_____

_____

_____

_____

_____

_____

_____

_____

_____

_____

Caring for you, the caregiver

~ Fortunately, my husband and I have always been content doing things round our home so "outside" therapy worked for us. The fact that Mom was never violent made things easier.
Myra's daughter, MN

~ I attend a men's Bible study group every Saturday morning and also a Wednesday morning renewal group. I work out at least twice a week at the health club.
Carol's husband, MN

~ Who had time? Who had the inclination to do that when someone else (my Mom) needed so very much care and time? No – I failed the Caring for Self – 101 class.
Genevieve's daughter, MN

~ I think my brother, sister and I supported each other. I always had someone to talk to and I think we saw "eye-to-eye". The decline was very sad, but we knew nothing could be done.
Mary's stepdaughter, MN

~ I barely take care of my own needs. There is not enough time in the day. I try to take care of my needs, but I can't. All of my needs are put on the back burner, so to speak.
Charlotte's daughter, TX

~ I saw the difficulty in self-care greatest in my Mom. She is a wonderfully selfless person who would do anything for anyone, especially her own mother. I had the advantage – and disadvantage – of being 1,800 miles away.   Gen's granddaughter, CA

~ I was only a part-time caregiver (three days every six weeks or so), so I was able to care for myself just fine. I don't have a "burned out" story like many [AD caregivers].
Helen's daughter, OR

~ I was consumed by mother's problems and disease and put aside my own needs (medical, social, etc.) and home affairs.
Helen's daughter, WA

~ We made a point to do things together. We included Mom sometimes as long as we could, but also did some things without her.
Donna's daughter, IA

~ I didn't have the daily burden so could "forget" and get on with my life. I dreaded visits to the nursing home when she was no longer responsive.
Mildred's daughter, IA

~ My life centered around Mom. Fortunately, I didn't suffer from any medical problems other than a blood-pressure issue. I think being 5 hours away, it was easy to "go on hold" after each phone call and put the situation out of my mind. Knitting needles also helped.

Matilda's daughter, MN

~ I went to the nursing home every day for the first year and became friends with other patients and their families. Then I cut back to every other day. Many times I would come home to be sick at my stomach. I started to get my life back.

Gerald's wife, IA

~ I try to get out and take time for myself. It is a challenge. I am also mother to a wonderful 3-year-old and wife to an awesome husband. As a family, we work together and live next door to my parents. So we care for them as they need it.

Roy's daughter, MN

~ Knowing that Lanie was in the hands of people who cared about her kept me from being depressed. My faith definitely kept me from falling apart.

Lanie's sister, MN

~ About two months after placing Reatha in the home, I became very depressed. I found a lady friend in a nearby town and we would see each other about twice a week. I told our son, who is a minister, about it and he almost disowned me. I see him maybe 3-4 times a year. My daughter doesn't like it, but she seems to understand the situation a little better.

Reatha's husband, IA

~ Mom visited Dad often. He was 25 miles away. She was very levelheaded about not going in bad weather. She had plenty of friends at the retirement home. Support was also there as other caregivers were there. I felt I had to watch out for my Mother at this time. Dad was taken care of. She needed the help more; I was more concerned about her.

Alvin's daughter, IA

~ I think Mom felt a certain sense of relief when Dad went to the nursing home and a tremendous load was lifted from her. Her health even improved.

Joe's daughter, IA

~ When Mother was living with us the second time, I would take her to the foster grandparents two times a week which was 15 miles each way. Sometimes, that really got to be a pain but it was something she really liked to do. Later at the nursing home, we continued this until the day care center had to close.

Margaret's daughter, KS

~ I did not do a good job of taking care of myself. For the most part, it was like if it wasn't something for Mom, it didn't exist for me. It was during this time that I also exhibited signs of anxiety so was put on Paxil to help – my doctor called it "situational depression". I started to feel better after that but still didn't get out and "do" for myself like I should have. I think the key to this is to accept that there is a limit as to what you can do for your loved one and try to live life for yourself, too. Easier said than done, most days.

Lanie's daughter, MN

YOUR THOUGHTS -

_____

_____

_____

_____

_____

_____

_____

_____

_____

_____

_____

_____

Only one type of worry is correct: to worry because you worry too much. (proverb)

Creative care and activities for the patient

~ Because so much has happened in the last year, as my Dad deteriorates and no longer is able to do so many things he once was able to do, I coordinate others in the family to do things. He enjoys fishing and we are attempting to get him out once a week to do this. Dad enjoys gardening but is limited physically. We try to get the older grandchildren to help there. Whenever Dad would like an outing, we try to get him out. It is so important to keep AD people active so they do not lose complete hope in living. Roy's daughter, MN

~ One day when I went to visit Lanie [in the nursing home], she was peeling some apples. That was the first time I found out how they tried to make the patients feel useful. That really boosted my morale and when Lanie said, "they make us work", I was on Cloud Nine! Lanie's sister, MN

~ The home had daily activities and being Mom was in the Special Care unit, she could go if someone escorted her. That worked perfect for me. My sister went mornings and I went afternoons. For a while, Mom enjoyed the flower garden the home had. We did have some nice times out there. Myra's daughter, MN

~ Carol enjoys going to the casinos. She went with her three sisters and our daughter to Las Vegas last winter. We go to the local casinos about once a month. I give her a money allotment and I gave our daughter the money for Carol to spend in Las Vegas. We go out to a restaurant every Thursday and, one Thursday a month, we take Carol's aunt and cousin with us. Carol seems to enjoy these outings. Everywhere we go, she shows people pictures of Max, her dog, and a picture of our great-grandson. I always just sit there and smile. Carol's husband, MN

~ Mom wasn't one to participate in very many activities. She would get involved at her church but there wasn't much outside of that. I remember the last time my husband and I took her out to eat. She could not remember how to use the silverware, could not order a meal, and had no idea of where we were. It was all terribly sad. Genevieve's daughter, MN

~ Alvin enjoyed going for a malt. I took him until it got hard to manage. I also took him cookies and candy bars. And he never forgot this. He always asked for them. Alvin's wife, IA

~ One of the treats that Mother loved to do was to go to garage sales. I think of her each time I go to one.
Margaret's daughter, KS

~ They played hymn tapes for her. If she was having a good day, social services would visit her and tell us about what she'd said or done.

Mildred's daughter, IA

~ There were many activities offered in the assisted living home. Mom participated in some and we all did if we were there.

Donna's daughter, IA

~ Mom enjoyed having her hair washed and set. She was also glad to have a permanent occasionally. While we did visit her often, we did not take her out for fear we could not get her back home.

Mary's daughter, MN

~ Even though Mom never admitted she liked the nursing home, we felt she was getting very good care. She had three good meals a day, she was clean and the staff was very dedicated to their job.

Matilda's daughter, MN

~ I never took Gerald out of the nursing home except for once, to go to the doctor, and I think that was easier for both of us. I was afraid I wouldn't be able to handle him, not be able to get him back into the car. He was pretty far gone by the time we placed him in the nursing home.

Gerald's wife, IA

~ I felt Mother could have participated in more activities in the home. Several times when I visited, there were musical or dancing programs which they did not bring her down to see. I complained about it but I don't think they wanted to bother with her. We continued to bring her to our homes every Sunday until she was afraid of the elevator [at the home] and it became impossible to get her in or out of the car, etc. She was more secure in the home.

Mary's stepdaughter, MN

~ Our family always visited regularly to provide consistency in routine. Grandma didn't always recognize the players, but the players were always there; the consistency seemed so important.

Gen's granddaughter, CA

~ Getting ice cream, taking a drive, looking at Christmas lights, playing bingo, watching Lucy programs. Helen's daughter, OR

~ When Mom was back in her home, her caregivers took her to concerts, played bingo and looked at pictures with her. I would take her to play bingo once a week.

Helen's daughter, WA

~ Once Mom entered the nursing home, she was enfolded in a structured day filled with exercise, treats, attention by staff, and "girly" stuff like nail care and makeup. I particularly got a kick out of Mom wearing nail polish as she had always maintained that she had ugly nails. Now, she was so proud of those pretty pink fingernails. My aunt and I continued to take her out for drives and treats – individually as long as we could and then together as a team when Mom got harder to physically manipulate.   Lanie's daughter, MN

YOUR THOUGHTS -

_____

_____

_____

_____

_____

_____

_____

_____

_____

_____

_____

_____

No one knows what he can do until he tries. (Publilius Syrus, *Moral Sayings*)

Extra journaling pages

WINTER – The Sad Reality

Symptoms of decline

~ Mother quit eating and drinking the early part of March. By April, she was no longer interested in getting out of bed. She lost her ability to swallow food and water. We were told that that part of the brain telling her this [how to swallow] was destroyed by the Alzheimer's.   Mary's daughter, MN

~ My sister received a call from the nursing home that Mom was unresponsive. My sister went to the home and Mom entered the hospital. She was very dehydrated, had pneumonia and had a case of the flu. My sister and I sat with her most of the days for almost two weeks. The day that she passed, we talked and both of us said "we didn't think Mom was going to make it through this illness". She passed away a little after midnight. She could no longer swallow any food or liquids.
                                                                                    Matilda's daughter, MN

~ Gerald walked less, slept more, fell a lot and walked into walls or fell out of chairs. He had a blank look, a sick look. He didn't seem to know I was there, holding his hand. He had to be fed.   Gerald's wife, IA

~ It got to the point that when I would visit Lanie in the home, she wouldn't acknowledge my presence. She just sat there and stared at people. The one thing that always made her react was when someone brought a pet in. She also reacted when someone would bring in a baby.   Lanie's sister, MN

~ Dad could always eat normally. His walking deteriorated the most.   Alvin's daughter, IA

~ Mother fell and broke her hip, but the doctor said after her operation that she broke her thigh bone, and that caused her to fall. She was in a lot of pain and they had to move her to change her Depends, to get her up to eat, etc. Margaret's daughter, KS

~ Mom twice lost the ability to swallow and then rebounded when we thought death was imminent.   Mildred's daughter, IA

~ Clarence got pneumonia in September. He could not eat, swallow, etc. and went downhill in a hurry.   Clarence's wife, SC

~ The last two months, swallowing became a bit problem for Mom and oxygen was needed.   Myra's daughter, MN

~ Mom developed pneumonia and coded [alarms sounded that called medical staff]. She was resuscitated. It was difficult to understand her then because of tubes. The second time she coded, she was in a coma.   Donna's daughter, IA

~ Unmistakable signs of decline began in December, 1999. At least Mom never had to worry about the possibility of the world collapsing at the turn of the century! The swallowing ability disappeared. She could no longer even drink that awful "thickened" liquid junk they were trying to give her. Forget the nutritional drink – it would no longer go down her throat but would instead dribble out the sides of her mouth and down her skinny little neck onto the sweatshirt she wore. She would have been mortified to know what was happening to her. Genevieve's daughter, MN

~ Mother stopped feeding herself. She also became less steady on her feet and had several falls. The home had a policy that you must be able to feed yourself. We were told we could let her starve or find a new home. We found her a new home. Mary's stepdaughter, MN

~ When my Grandma had trouble swallowing, we had to face the issue of inserting a feeding tube. We knew she'd <u>never</u> want that, so, in respect of her wishes, we declined. Shortly thereafter, she develop pneumonia, likely the result of swallowing difficulty. We had to decide to treat or not treat the resultant pneumonia – a vicious circle, for certain. Gen's granddaughter, CA

~ Mom was no longer verbal and just rocked in her chair. She refused all intake and had to be syringe-fed. Her eventual death was pneumonia, probably caused by aspirating liquid into her lungs. It was no one's fault – it just happened. Helen's daughter, OR

~ Mom started to show an inability and disinterest in eating. It was as if she forgot how to eat. She had confusion about how to correctly use utensils. She was initially receptive to taking chocolate protein smoothies but later refused them. Swallowing seemed difficult for her. Helen's daughter, WA

~ Mom's ability to swallow began to decline after a bout with pneumonia. Because it was thought that the pneumonia was caused by liquids being swallowed incorrectly and aspirated into her lungs, all of her liquids were thickened before being served to her. Nothing like thick coffee to help the appetite . . . She began to have trouble with solids about 4 weeks before she died and it got to the point where she would not eat, even for me. Lanie's daughter, MN

YOUR THOUGHTS -

_____

_____

_____

_____

_____

_____

_____

_____

_____

_____

_____

_____

A special place in heaven is reserved for those who can weep but cannot pray. (proverb)

More medical decisions

~ My sister wanted to do a feeding tube. I flatly said no. I had to get my sister to start thinking about what Mom would want, not what she wanted.   Helen's daughter, OR

~ The in-home caregivers resigned and we placed Mom in the Adult Family Home where she had been previously. At that point, she was immobile and ate very little. After a month, she was hospitalized with aspiration pneumonia and died two days later. I had to honor Mom's Living Will which specified no feeding tube or respirator.   Helen's daughter, WA

~ We had to make decisions as to approving a DNR [order] or not. Two of us were in favor and one took longer to agree but finally did.   Donna's daughter, IA

~ We had DNR on Mom's record. The end came unexpectedly. She had a slight cold and staff found she had died when they did a bed check in the early morning.   Mildred's daughter, IA

~ They tried a feeding tube for water, but Mother continually pulled it out. I had to make the decision to discontinue this tube. That caused me much distress. **Author's note:** In a conversation, Mary's daughter also commented on how hard it was to handle the "you should . . ." comments from well-meaning people who had their own ideas about what to do for the AD patient.   Mary's daughter, MN

~ At a brief hospitalization, they wanted to insert a feeding tube. The Alzheimer's Association had their offices at this hospital so I went down and they helped strengthen me to say no to the feeding tube.   Gerald's wife, IA

~ Hospice took over when Clarence went to the nursing home and kept in contact with me and our daughter. Clarence's wife, SC

~ All decisions and steps were in place to keep Mom comfortable.   Myra's daughter, MN

~ The dreaded discussion took place. I was called in for a conference – the subject being Hospice care and the possibility of surgically implanting a feeding tube. Thank God, my Mom and I had the end-of-life discussions through the years. I knew she would never want a feeding tube to prolong her life. (What life? What quality of life was left at this point?) It was an easy decision for me to make – YES to Hospice care; an absolute NO to the feeding tube.   Genevieve's daughter, MN

~ The Cognex was discontinued. Her teeth needed care – some molars even fell out. We let it go as she would never let a dentist work on her and felt a general anesthetic would be too hard on her. Mary's stepdaughter, MN

~ Mom had a DNR [Do Not Resuscitate] order for Dad before entering the home. Alvin's daughter, IA

~ Dad's family [by genetics] has a negative reaction to most meds/drugs. When the cancer was found, very near his end, they put [medicinal] patches on him that put him in an unconscious state. Once removed, he returned but then was in pain again, so they were replaced and he just slept away. Joe's daughter, IA

~ From the point after her operation, she wanted to die and said so quite often. She was given pain pills, but it didn't seem to help. Margaret's daughter, KS

~ As Mom continued to be unable to eat or drink, the head nurse of the AD unit confirmed with me that my decision against inserting a feeding tube was still in place. She also gave me a heads-up that it was time to call hospice in. Hospice came in for a consultation on pain management and a new bed on a Thursday. Mom started hospice care on Friday and died the following Monday.

Lanie's daughter, MN

YOUR THOUGHTS -

The trip is never too hard if you know you are going home. (proverb)

Accepting that the end is near

~ Mom was in a coma for several days. At this point, we all wanted her to be free of all the pain and have peace. The doctors were pretty direct as to what was happening.   Donna's daughter, IA

~ My sister struggled with letting Mom go even until two days before Mom died. She wanted feeding tubes and treatment for pneumonia. But we talked and she finally decided that those measures were more for her, not Mom. Helen's daughter, OR

~ I had difficulties honoring my mother's living will but my sister insisted that we honor Mom's wishes. I felt like I was giving up on her.   Helen's daughter, WA

~ When hospice became involved, I was wore out. I had made 25 seventy-mile trips to see Clarence. The daughter and I went to see him most of the day on October 11, 2003. On the way home, we received a call on the cell phone that Clarence had passed away about 15 minutes after we left.   Clarence's wife, SC

~ Very few words are spoken but I hold her hands and tell her I love her and that soon, "Mom, you'll be with Fritz again". Several times, her priest would come and pray with us.   Myra's daughter, MN

~ Acceptance of the end was "forced" upon me when I got a call telling me to come to the nursing home as quickly as possible. We arrived within ten minutes, as did four of my five children. My mother was nearly comatose at this point. We called a priest – I knew she would want this – and he administered Last Rites (for the second time) and prayed for her.   Genevieve's daughter, MN

~ Mother lived at the new residence for 18 months. They fed her. She walked, but falls became more common. One day, the physician's assistant called and said Mom's condition was stable. The next day, she called stating mother had just had a seizure. Mother was not alert and could not swallow. I chose to have her on seizure medicine and morphine to help her breathing and keep her comfortable. She lived nine more days. We knew the end was near. I was threatened and relieved.   Mary's stepdaughter, MN

~ I was getting worn out both physically and emotionally. Of course I felt relief when she died. It was her time. All for the better – my mom was gone before she died.   Marie's daughter, MN

~ I cried more tears when he was living than I did when he was "taken home". It was harder placing him in the nursing home. *Alvin's wife, IA*

~ We knew that the end would bring relief for him and us and that he would have no more suffering. *Joe's daughter, IA*

~ Because she didn't take any other medication and basically was healthy as a horse, I believe she decided not to eat and to shut her system down. She was given a nutritional drink every few hours. *Margaret's daughter, KS*

~ We had prayed for her peaceful passing. Very easy to accept. *Mildred's daughter, IA*

~ My sister and I realized the end was near. All we wanted was for her to be with our Dad. *Matilda's daughter, MN*

~ My pastor was out of town – REALLY out – in India for four weeks. Gerald was in final stages and I do believe he waited for her to return. She got back on a Monday night, came to the nursing home at 11:00 a.m. on Tuesday and Gerald died at noon. *Gerald's wife, IA*

~ My niece and I were at Lanie's bedside during the last few hours of her life. This might sound hard, but I kept praying silently for God to take her and thanked him so much when he finally did. *Lanie's sister, MN*

~ By the time hospice was involved, I was worn out physically and emotionally. All I wanted for her was some peace and I believed that dying would give that to her. I probably came across to some as hard, but I only felt a sense of relief that she was finally at the end of her journey.

Lanie's daughter, MN

YOUR THOUGHTS -

From happiness to sorrow takes a moment; from sorrow to happiness takes years (proverb)

Hospice help

~ They were so kind and understanding that you would almost think it was their loved one in that bed.   Lanie's sister, MN

~ Hospice is a great help to all. They still keep in touch with me to see how I am doing.   Clarence's wife, SC

~ Hospice was akin to a band of angels sent to earth for the sole reason of comfort for Mom and emotional support for me and for my family. They flew in on angel wings and pretty much set things in motion. We only needed Hospice care for about 10 days, but they continued their follow-up for an entire year after my Mom's death.   Genevieve's daughter, MN

~ We are very grateful for the care and ongoing concern Hospice offered my family. They even offered on-going counseling after Grandma passed away, especially concerned with my niece and nephews (her great-grandchildren). Hospice was one of the best interventions for my Grandma and for my family. I can't say enough about their merits.   Gen's granddaughter, CA

Author's note about hospice: It surprised me that very few of the caregivers who contributed anecdotes to this book took advantage of the services that hospice offers. A few things to consider about hospice:

1. Hospice services are generally paid for by Medicare and other insurances. Hospice representatives are very clear about where the money is coming from so that families understand that it will not be an additional financial burden.

2. Hospice works with the nursing home or personal caregivers to give the AD patient <u>additional</u> care and comfort. This can be particularly worthwhile to the family and/or personal caregivers – it reassures them that the AD patient is getting the attention that will ensure as much emotional and physical relief as possible.

3. Services are generally offered when the patient has been diagnosed as having 6 months or less to live. This timeframe may give a caregiver pause because it means accepting another sign of the AD patient's decline. It's important to remember that hospice is about the comfort of the <u>patient</u>. This may be one more thing for a caregiver to have to work through, emotionally, but the loved one will certainly benefit (and, ultimately, so will the caregiver).

4. Hospice offers wonderful follow-up services which can be very comforting to the caregiver(s). After the strain of giving so much to someone else, there can be a letdown after the funeral, etc. The caregiver's informal support group may very well be ready to move on, but the grief is often still very real for the family/caregiver. Hospice is very willing to listen and counsel, even months after the loss. They are trained to do this, and they do it well.

~ Hospice was wonderful, even for the short time that we had their assistance. They brought in a different bed with more positions that would help keep Mom comfortable and prescribed meds that would keep her from feeling any pain as she slowly wasted away. They also offered good follow-up care to me – phone calls and letters on a regular basis for some time after Mom died.

Lanie's daughter, MN

Where love is, no room is too small.. (proverb)

YOUR THOUGHTS -

_____

_____

_____

_____

_____

_____

_____

_____

_____

_____

_____

_____

Faith-based comfort

~ After her hip surgery in the hospital, our parish priest gave her the Last Rites. My brother, myself and some others were there during the service. Then she went to the nursing home – 3 days later she died.   Marie's daughter, MN

~ We were raised in the church. We had a great faith that carried us through.   Alvin's daughter, IA

~ Mom died at night. One of the nurses at the nursing home was sitting and holding her hand when she died. Worst phone call I ever had. Thanks to the nursing home, we made her funeral arrangements in advance which saved us more stress.   Mary's daughter, MN

~ Mom died at the hospital. Neither my sister or I were there. A nurse had finished giving Mom some meds and turned her onto her side. The nurse finished her rounds and when she walked by Mom's room, noticed Mom wasn't breathing. The nursing home that Mom was in had a death prayer, which is attended by the staff. I'm not sure the hospital where Mom died has such a routine.   Matilda's daughter, MN

~ I will always remember staff in a circle around Gerald's bed – crying and caring. And the nursing home staff bringing me food those last two days or taking me/making me go out for fresh air and to get a away a little.   Gerald's wife, IA

~ After receiving Last Rites, Mom suddenly sat up in bed, reached out her arms and smiled. Her face looked peaceful and content and she kept her eyes on a point of the wall where her outstretched arms were pointing. I don't know exactly what she saw – but I know she saw something. Whether it was an angel, Mary, the face of God, my father, her Mom, I'll never know exactly what, but the vision brought great peace to her. After about 30 seconds, she lay back down and lapsed into a coma. She had developed pneumonia at this point: she spiked a high fever and her breathing became extremely labored. Shortly before my mother died, my daughter and I were discussing a visit from another daughter and her three children. They were expected to arrive within the hour. We don't really know if people in a coma hear us, but at this time, my mother's breathing became a bit stronger. When the children arrived, they all kissed her, touched her arm and talked to her. I will always swear that she waited until she could hear those great-grandchildren in her room before she died: she died within 10 minutes of their arrival - on January 2, 2000 at about 2:00 p.m. We were all very comforted by what happened tha day.   Genevieve's daughter, MN

~ Mother received the Sacrament of the Sick. A friend from church came and said the rosary at her bedside; I prayed at her bedside.

Mary's stepdaughter, MN

~ I take comfort in knowing my family was with my Grandma when she passed away. Even though I was not with them, they were in my heart.

Gen's granddaughter, CA

~ While Mom was in the hospital, she received the Sacrament of the Anointing of the Sick from a priest and he prayed for her. It was comforting to me although she was probably incoherent at the time as she was on morphine.

Helen's daughter, WA

~ Father John came in to see Clarence every day in the nursing home and was there with us a few minutes before Clarence died. Clarence always smiled and held out his hand to shake hands with him.

Clarence's wife, SC

~ Several times, Mom's priest would come and pray with us.

Myra's daughter, MN

~ The most touching thing re: faith-based comfort occurred just after Mom died in the nursing home. Available staff gathered around her bed and shared how they remembered her on a personal level and prayed for her.   Lanie's daughter, MN

YOUR THOUGHTS –

_____

_____

_____

_____

_____

_____

_____

_____

_____

_____

_____

_____

_____

When dust returns to the earth, the spirit shall return to God, who gave it.

(Bible, *Ecclesiastes 12:7*)

The worst thing about this death

~ We weren't with her when she died.

Mildred's daughter, IA

~ Although Mom had been lost to us months in advance, her death was still a shock and left me with an empty feeling.

Mary's daughter, MN

~ We were all tired of Mom being unhappy or sick and wished it was over. When she did pass away, I wanted her back. I wasn't ready for her to die. Except for the last two weeks, she did have some good days.

Matilda's daughter, MN

~ I had learned: they are not dying because they are not eating; they are not eating because they are dying. I honestly think they know and choose not to eat at that time.

Gerald's wife, IA

~ I guess I thought that when Lanie finally passed away, she would have a peaceful look on her face. Instead, her mouth was open and her lips curved down, as if still in pain.

Lanie's sister, MN

~ Knowing Clarence was dying and could not eat or drink was hard to take. He had lost 45 pounds in three months.

Clarence's wife, SC

~ The worst thing for me is that Dad suffered (unnecessarily) for so long before anyone discovered the cancer and knew that the physical pain existed. I feel that as a caregiver myself, I should have noticed this as well as the nursing home personnel.

Joe's daughter, IA

~ I did not get to see Mom before she died. Although she probably would not have known I was there, she died without any family present. I should have left home sooner, having only missed her by 30 minutes. I do feel guilty about that. I should have come the day before but perhaps I was in denial myself, because I thought she would recover from the pneumonia.

Helen's daughter, OR

~ I had gone back to Iowa after five days of watching her in a coma. We had agreed on DNR if Mom coded [went into failure that required a hospital team to attend to her immediately]. I was home on Monday and went to work the next day. On Wednesday morning, I got the call that Mom had passed away. She had pneumonia and congestive heart disease. Pneumonia was the cause of death.

Donna's daughter, IA

~ I hated to see her die after a 13 year struggle and knowing she would have hated to die this way. Mary's stepdaughter, MN

~ My Grandma developed a pneumonia as a result of her inability to properly swallow. My family could have been aggressive in treating the pneumonia and Grandma may have recovered. The cycle was undoubtedly repetitive – the decisions endless. I admire the strength and courage of my family to truly respect my grandmother's wishes and regard them above our own fear of losing her.   Gen's granddaughter, CA

~ The very worst thing was watching her suffer with the terribly high fever and watching her chest rise and fall with each difficult breath. I was constantly with her from Thursday evening until her death on Sunday afternoon. I would wet a washcloth with cool water, put it on her head, and within a minute, the cloth was no longer cool and needed to be changed. I'm not certain how high the fever became – the sheets and pillowcase needed changing very often – but it was horrible to watch her suffer. My Mom always hated her hands – the fingers were skinny and on the backs of her hands, the veins were a visible blue color. Her hands were on top of the sheets and all I could think of was the beautiful items those hands produced during her lifetime. She used to knit, embroider, crochet, sew and do tatting, needlepoint, china painting and many other things. I hope she knows now that her "ugly" hands weren't so ugly after all. I did take a couple of photos of her hands as she was dying and these photos are very precious to me.
                     Genevieve's daughter, MN

~ The worst thing for me was knowing that Mom was dying because she couldn't eat or drink. Starvation and dehydration are so fundamentally preventable and yet, her body could not accommodate the means to avoid them. It was so hard to watch her skin pull up over her bones. Some months before, Mom had had an episode (unresponsive, uneven breathing) that prompted the head nurse of the AD unit to call me to get there <u>now</u>, but Mom quickly rebounded from that one. This time, the final outcome was certain.

Lanie's daughter, MN

YOUR THOUGHTS -

_____

_____

_____

_____

_____

_____

_____

_____

_____

_____

What is it that troubles you? Death? Who lives forever? (Samuel Ha-Nagid)

The best thing about this death

~ I was at her bedside

Marie's daughter, MN

~ Seeing Mom at peace was wonderful. The funeral directors were able to make her look so nice that we were able to have an open-casket funeral.

Mildred's daughter, IA

~ My children came home as often as they could and of course, came for the funeral. Our granddaughter, who was 4 at the time, asked at the meal if we were "celebrating Grandpa today". What a way to put it!

Alvin's daughter, IA

~ The nurse told us Mom just stopped breathing. She didn't feel Mom had struggled at all.

Matilda's daughter, MN

~ Gerald just quit breathing, gently and peacefully. I had cried for almost 10 years through this journey so this was a relief that it was over. I had lost him bit-by-bit.

Gerald's wife, IA

~ Lanie was finally at rest.

Lanie's sister, MN

~ Clarence quit breathing and passed away very peacefully.

Clarence's wife, SC

~ Mom was well prepared. We said our good-byes. We thank God for all her years of love and realize her painful journey is past. She died on August 26, 2002 at 10:14.

Myra's daughter, MN

~ I knew Mom was a woman of faith and she believed that God was good and would watch over those she had to leave behind. She believed in the afterlife and I know she watches over us from above. We now have seven grandchildren and I know she sees them and asks God's blessings for them as well.

Genevieve's daughter, MN

~ I felt relief that the struggle was over. I couldn't see joy in her life for about five years. She was a religious woman and I felt she was finally home.

Mary's stepdaughter, MN

~ I was not present at the time of my grandmother's death. I'd returned to California only days prior. I still struggle about my decision to return home. At the time, once again the prognosis was uncertain and I'd already used up all of my paid time off – dang . . . Work was a necessary reality.

Gen's granddaughter, CA

~ Mom's suffering is over. She went peacefully, the morphine having done its job and demands on my sister are less (but still estate/probate to come).   Helen's daughter, OR

~ It was a relief that she wasn't suffering anymore since her life had become a struggle.   Helen's daughter, WA

~ We all certainly felt she was in a better place and were glad for her. She hadn't been "our Mom" for the last year.
                                                                                                    Donna's daughter, IA

~ I was relieved when the angels came. The worst is seeing their deterioration and the helplessness of the situation. Our daughters and I were at his side when he died.   Alvin's wife, IA

~ We were all with her when she died peacefully at our home. She went to sleep, her heart stopped and she quit breathing. Her prayers came true. God took her home to be with Dad.   Milta's son, KS

~ We were called about 4:00 in the morning to say that Mother had passed on and she had died quietly in her sleep.
                                                                                                    Margaret's daughter, KS

~ She just quit breathing so it was very peaceful. To quote the obituary that I wrote for her: "[She was] released from the scourge of Alzheimer's to fly freely with the angels." The sense of this being the best thing for her was so strong that all I felt at the time was a sense of relief for her. My sense of loss was long over – she had been "gone" for months prior to her death.

Lanie's daughter, MN

YOUR THOUGHTS -

_____

_____

_____

_____

_____

_____

_____

_____

_____

_____

_____

_____

Death is merely moving from one home to another. (proverb)

_____

_____

_____

_____

_____

_____

_____

_____

_____

_____

_____

_____

_____

_____

_____

_____

In memoriam: the service of remembrance

~ All the children and grandchildren and great-grands were there. We opened the full casket as some wondered where his feet were!

Alvin's wife, IA

~ Dad had stated his desire to be cremated very early on (years earlier). His remains were buried in Rosehill Cemetery.

Joe's daughter, IA

~ She was cremated in KC and we had a memorial service for her at our Lutheran church in Shawnee. Then our whole family took her back to Tucson to be interred with Dad.

Milta's son, KS

~ We would play Anne Murray's CD and one song was "Amazing Grace" and Mother said, "I would like to have her sing that at my funeral." So, via a tape, Anne Murray sang at Mother's funeral. She would have been pleased. Many people came to the funeral – even the coordinator from Foster Grandparents.

Margaret's daughter, KS

~ It was a wonderful celebration of Mom's life. Many people spoke to us of her part in their lives.

Mildred's daughter, IA

~ Our pastor did a wonderful service and much to my surprise, weeks after the service, we were still getting calls telling us how impressed they were with the service.

Mary's daughter, MN

~ My sister and I made arrangements for Mom's funeral. We chose a beautiful casket and a lavender dress that she had worn to my niece's wedding. She looked so peaceful. My Mom's nephew (Mom's favorite) did the funeral service. All of Mom's children (and spouses), grandchildren and great-grandchildren attended the funeral service and burial.

Matilda's daughter, MN

~ I had Gerald cremated and there was a memorial service at our church.

Gerald's wife, IA

~ We were sad but not sorry at Dad's passing. He was now free. Placing him in a home was far worse. There are worse things than death.

Alvin's daughter, IA

~ The memorial service was beautiful and it left me with a wonderful feeling. It was so nice to see some of Lanie's friends from way back.

Lanie's sister, MN

~ At Mom's request, we had her cremated.

Donna's daughter, IA

~ We had a memorial service in the Methodist church in Port Royal and a viewing at an undertaker in Beaufort. We flew Clarence's body to Millville, PA and had a viewing at an undertaker there and funeral services the following day. After the funeral, a local Methodist church had dinner for all who attended the services. Clarence's wife, SC

~ We had a funeral Mass at the church my mother attended since 1938. It was peaceful and she would have loved the music. Mom requested a closed coffin because "nobody needs to stare at me and say how awful I look". I am so glad I decided to have the casket opened prior to the funeral. I've since learned through grief counseling how important it is to actually see the body. The grandchildren placed drawings and photos in the casket for Grandma and this provided comfort to them as well. I think Mom has forgiven me for not following her direction this one time. By opening the coffin, we also unwittingly opened a can of worms within the family. (My God, I should not have used the word "worms" in this context!). Anyway, the controversy was over the dress. After the funeral, we were sitting and discussing the day when I mentioned the "periwinkle" [blue] dress my mother wore for her burial. My cousins and one of my daughters – in unison – said, "Periwinkle? It was purple!" It's become an ongoing family joke now whether the dress was periwinkle or purple. Yes, there can be funny things at funerals, too. Genevieve's daughter, MN

~ We returned Mother to Superior and she was buried from her childhood church, laid to rest next to my Dad. Despite being gone for so many years, many friends and relatives attended the funeral. That was comforting.
  Mary's stepdaughter, MN

~ I still have violet plants from my Grandma's funeral. They were brought to my Mom by a former work colleague. I don't know if that colleague knew of my Grandma's affection for violets, but maintaining these plants offers me a daily reconnection with my Grandma. When the plants bloom, I feel her presence and always feel her ongoing guidance. Though her last few months were of mental decline, the Grandma I remember, the one that guides and advises me even today, well, she's fully herself as I knew her when I was a very young child. Gen's granddaughter, CA

~ There was a regular Catholic Mass in Mom's memory. I gave a speech in which I injected lots of humor and heart. Only family and caregivers attended (along with the regular congregation). Helen's daughter, OR

~ We had the same funeral service in the same church where my Dad's funeral service had been. We selected the same casket for her that she had selected for my Dad 3 years earlier. She was buried next to him. Helen's daughter, WA

~ I had Mom cremated and we held a memorial service at the same funeral home our family always uses. My son and his wife drove up from Tennessee even though they had just done the same trip two weeks prior because <u>her</u> grandma unexpectedly died. My daughter, son-in-law and grandson were also there and my grandson, aged 18 months, entertained the group just by being a toddler – Mom would have enjoyed that. Many former neighbors and friends attended. A hospice chaplain gave the homily and did a fine job except for mispronouncing Mom's full name (Ralane). It was fitting, in a way, because her whole life, people always mispronounced it. In one last "should have", I should have had him use her nickname – Lanie.

Lanie's daughter, MN

YOUR THOUGHTS -

_____

_____

_____

_____

_____

_____

_____

_____

_____

_____

Sympathy is a little medicine to soothe the ache in another's heart. (proverb)

Tying up the loose ends

~ This was all done when Dad died in 2000. Everything in Mom's room, except for photos, was donated to the nursing home.   Mildred's daughter, IA

~ We donated most of the things Mom had at the nursing home to the nursing home, i.e. lift chair and clothes. It's amazing how few things some of the residents have, even in a small community.   Matilda's daughter, MN

~ I had intended to scatter ashes on the golf course at our country club but didn't. I'm glad I waited. For his Eagle Scout project, a young man is putting in a Memorial Garden at our church so this is where Gerald will be later this summer [2004].   Gerald's wife, IA

~ The final farewell came when we scattered Lanie's ashes in Lake Superior at Duluth. We might have shut the door on her life, but she would never be shut out of our memories.   Lanie's sister, MN

~ Clarence's estate is in probate because his will was notarized, but didn't have the two witness signatures that are required here. It takes eight months to end it.   Clarence's wife, SC

~ I still have some things in boxes from my mother's apartment that I can't bring myself to open. It's just not the right time. That time will present itself – I've learned not to push it before I'm ready to deal with it.   Genevieve's daughter, MN

~ Furniture, etc. was donated to the home. Her valuables were divided among the five children.   Mary's stepdaughter, MN

~ I immediately washed all of her clothes and they went to Goodwill. Then I cleaned her house from top to bottom. She always kept a clean house and it seemed a fitting tribute to get her house in order, the way she would want it to look. Closing out everything else is still ongoing; the burden is borne by my sister who had Power of Attorney. Helen's daughter, OR

~ We donated her clothes to charity. I am now in the middle of probating the will.   Helen's daughter, WA

~ I lived in the family home until I sold it two years after Mom died.   Marie's daughter, MN

~ The funeral home took care of the arrangements to have Mother's body flown to Minnesota. However, it first went to Atlanta. We drove up [to MN] on Friday and the body didn't get there until early evening.   Margaret's daughter, KS

~ I opted to sprinkle her ashes at a later date (from a boat into Lake Superior in the summer of 2003 with both of her sisters present). I donated her chair and dresser to the nursing home, her clothes to Goodwill and took other things home to sort out later. I notified the County that she was gone and we settled up financially with the nursing home. We'd scaled her life down to such a level that I was able to close things out very efficiently.   Lanie's daughter, MN

When you must, you can. (proverb)

YOUR THOUGHTS -

_____

_____

_____

_____

_____

_____

_____

_____

_____

_____

_____

_____

_____

Moving forward with grieving

~ After the funeral, I kind of fell apart. With all of the responsibility gone, I felt out of control Went to a psychiatrist who pu
me on Prozac and after a time, I felt much better and got a new part-time job. Marie's daughter, MN

~ I had already gone through the grief stages. Alvin's wife, IA

~ I think we all had grieved as Mom lost her ability to recognize us so few tears were shed. I have some remorse about my
father's death because we had some unsettled issues. I didn't feel he allowed any of us to do some things that would have
made their final years easier. I didn't feel he ever understood her dementia; he seemed to feel she was willfully making his
life harder. Dad died in October of 2000. My oldest brother, who was an alcoholic and ne'er-do-well, died in February,
2003. I will always feel my folks' caring for him and his many problems contributed to Mom's problems and decline. Mildred's daughter, IA

~ I am still grieving my Mom's death (she passed away 12-16-03). We are in the process of selling her house and her
belongings. I am still wondering why we are doing it. I have called Mom's phone number and the operator informed me
that the number had been disconnected and I have also visited the nursing home and someone else is in her room. Matilda's daughter, MN

~ My grieving was done when Lanie was alive. I didn't have to make any adjustments after her death. Lanie's sister, MN

~ I attended a grief group offered by a local funeral home. I was fortunate because there was an excellent facilitator – Dick
Obershaw. He is an nationally-known counselor and really brought things into perspective for me. He had excellent ideas
and many words of comfort for those of us attending the sessions. I will always be thankful for this opportunity to move
beyond the grief and slowly, slowly back into the tasks of everyday life. Genevieve's daughter, MN

~ I missed going to the home and feeding Mom. It was the only thing I could do for her and I enjoyed it. I missed her even ir
her sickness but was relieved it was over. Mary's stepdaughter, MN

~ At the time of my grandmother's death, I was in California. I was on a flight home within hours of hearing of her death. I was glad to be home during such an emotionally trying time for my family. I was able to provide strength in decisions regarding Grandma's funeral. The funeral home seemed to correlate our love for Grandma with the amount we spent on her funeral – an abomination in my mind. We selected what my grandmother would have wanted, in spite of pressures to spend more to "better glorify her memory". We did what my grandmother wanted. Gen's granddaughter, CA

~ Mostly, I was done grieving by the time Mom died. A piece of her died each time I saw her. Truth be told, I was relieved. Caring for her those last few months had been very difficult as her physical abilities declined rapidly.

Helen's daughter, OR

~ My Dad died suddenly which was more traumatic since it was unexpected whereas, with my mother, we recognized that the AD was the beginning of the end.

Helen's daughter, WA

~ My Dad died suddenly and I didn't have the chance to gradually get used to the idea that he was going to die like I did with Mom. I found that by the time she did die, I had pretty much gone through all of the recognized stages of grief – Denial, Anger, Bargaining, Depression and Acceptance.

Lanie's daughter, MN

YOUR THOUGHTS -

_____

_____

_____

_____

_____

_____

_____

_____

_____

_____

_____

_____

The song is ended, but the melody lingers on. (Irving Berlin, lyric)

Moving forward with life – you, the caregiver

~ We often talk about Mother, remembering the funny things she would say or do, but always with a fondness and a smile.

Margaret's daughter, KS

~ My brother and I were able to settle the estate in a very amiable manner with our older, more needy brother already deceased. I was sad that Mom became so awful-looking as her dementia took its course. Sometimes the great-grandchildren were afraid of her and her noisy chanting. It also caused fellow nursing home residents to resent her. Mildred's daughter, IA

~ We took care of Mom since my dad died in 1969. With her gone, we find we have lots of time on our hands.

Mary's daughter, MN

~ I am still working on "moving forward".

Matilda's daughter, MN

~ There is life after Alzheimer's!! I have found that volunteering for Alzheimer's is very fulfilling. I like the phrase – **It Is Never Too Late To Be What You Might Have Been**. I love giving speeches about AD and letting people know about this disease. I have a good life, active in church, play lots of bridge, belong to a discussion group, do line dancing, etc. I walk two miles every day.

Gerald's wife, IA

~ The one good thing that came from this whole thing is the strong love and friendship that developed with my niece. I knew who she was from the day she was born, but I never <u>knew</u> her.

Lanie's sister, MN

~ As only a part-time caregiver, the impact was not great. I am relieved to not have to travel so many miles every few weeks. I struggled with "I should have known" and "I should have seen" thoughts that suggest that we could have understood sooner. The good news is that nothing bad happened while the family was figuring this out. I struggle with "I should have been more aware/sensitive" and "I was too selfish". I also think about things like whether children should be taking in their AD parents or is it OK to put them in an AD facility, because that's the best place for them. Helen's daughter, OR

~ Mom had a very complicated estate which has been very time-consuming to settle. Because of this, I have not been able to resume a normal life as of yet.

Helen's daughter, WA

~ I had full support of family and friends. I did not have to make a move after Alvin died. I didn't need to make major changes.

Alvin's wife, IA

~ I'm a stronger person for having been able to accompany my mother through the progress of her awful disease. I understand more fully how fragile and precious life really is. One's world can be turned upside down in an instant. I've learned to appreciate my life and everyone in it each and every day. I keep reminding myself to take nothing for granted. I also know I can deal with whatever life throws my way. It has deepened my faith in God: not in the confines of the church of my youth, but in everyday things such as family, friends, nature, quiet, a good joke, a wonderful book, and on and on. Who knew that out of anguish can come peace if you only open your heart to accept it.

Genevieve's daughter, MN

~ I don't feel I really grieved [at the end]. I lost my Mom many years earlier and death was a relief. Mary's stepdaughter, MN

~ My Mom, my brother and sisters, and I have always shared a special bond. I am hoping that the closeness of her children has eased my Mom's feeling of responsibility as an "only child". My grandparents were such an integral part of my childhood. Grieving the deaths of both my grandfather and my grandmother was equivalent to me as losing a parent.

Gen's granddaughter, CA

~ I started biking and golfing with friends. I had severe acid reflux and have had to be on medication. There was a lot of tension in the pit of my stomach. BUT – I would do it again. Shortly after my Mother died, I took her sister who had Alzheimer's out every Sunday. My aunt has since died so now, for the last two years, I take my sister who also has Alzheimer's, out once a week to relieve my brother-in-law. He does a remarkable job caring for her. Her kids want her in a nursing home, but he "wants his honey at home" after 50 years of marriage.

Marie's daughter, MN

~ I was lucky in that my close relationship with my aunt, which was forged during Mom's illness, continued. My children and friends continue their support and graciously remember Mom with me. I found that there was so much I wanted to do that I had a hard time focusing on starting anything: I just wasn't used to doing for myself. A year and a half after Mom died, though, I did write a book - with help from some very caring people - in the hope that our experiences will help other AD caregivers!

Lanie's daughter, MN

YOUR THOUGHTS -

Everything that grows begins small and becomes big.
But grief starts big and becomes small – and disappears. (Ibn Gabirol)

_____

_____

_____

_____

_____

_____

_____

_____

_____

_____

_____

_____

_____

Things you learned about yourself during this AD journey

~ I learned I can be patient when I want to, when I really need to, as there is no profit in losing patience with someone who no longer has the capacity to understand what is going on around them. I learned that I don't seem to grieve as much/like others. I wonder if this is an indication that I don't get close to people like others do. I learned that I am afraid of AD, afraid that my husband will have to become a caregiver, afraid I will become the same angry woman my mother became.

Helen's daughter, OR

~ I learned that I have the will and determination to not give up and the ability to deal with difficult situations.

Helen's daughter, WA

~ I was gone a lot after High School. My relationship with Mother was peaceful but not close. I was too flamboyant at times and couldn't talk about myself and her. In her early stages, she would tell everyone "I don't know what I would do without Mary Ann" which made me feel good.

Marie's daughter, MN

~ I believe that the short experience we had with my mother helped a lot when my wife's mother came to live with us, and we had to deal with her AD.

Milta's son, KS

~ I regret that I didn't talk to her more about her relatives and her feelings about different things. Maybe it is the "Swedish" thing to not let emotions show. I believe she is in a better place without pain but with the Lord and all of the family that has gone on before her.

Margaret's daughter, KS

~ I always felt Mom had reverted to a small child who wondered what she was being punished for by being taken from her home.

Mildred's daughter, IA

~ I wish I would have had more patience with Mom during her lifetime. We were not with Mom when she passed away. I feel bad that she died alone. My husband is a good listener. Otherwise, I don't have anyone close that I can vent with. The support group has been a wonderful help.

Matilda's daughter, MN

~ I learned what a blessing siblings can be. We grieved for years together. We supported each other and made decisions together. That made it much easier.

Mary's stepdaughter, MN

~ I sometimes regret that I wasn't willing for Gerald to find a place in Florida for us to winter as he loved Florida and loved golf. I was stubborn – but also think I was right as everything would have been harder if we had moved away – harder for me, anyhow. I think I did the best I could. I wish our daughter would have been more involved and closer to me, but I understand – it was my job, my commitment.

Gerald's wife, IA

~ I learned, to an extent, to accept the things I cannot change. It's as simple as that. Also, I thank God every day for my health which gives me the opportunity to enjoy life to its fullest.

Lanie's sister, MN

~ Living alone and taking care of everything for 2 ½ months helped me after Clarence died. It's rough living alone, but friends from church and neighbors help a lot.

Clarence's wife, SC

~ I've learned I'm stronger than I thought I was, that there is more to life than worrying about how fat I look on a particular day, that I will never measure up to my idea of perfection, that I'll never be a size 4, so quit trying. I hug people a bit more tightly, I smile more, and I hold my family and friends closely within my heart and treasure them even more. I look for the good in people because you never know what they are going through in their personal lives. I have a long way to go, but I think I'm a better person for having gone on this journey. I pray more for peace in the world because the photos of families being torn apart before their time due to wars, famine, etc. bring heartache and tears to my eyes at each newscast. All in all, my journey was a learning experience and one that now has me praying for the doctors doing research on AD and the other horrible diseases.

Genevieve's daughter, MN

~ Because I lived so far away, I'd always wished I could be there more. On the other hand, so much of my day-to-day life reminds me of my grandmother that I feel as though I've never left her fond embrace. It is her enduring love and kindness that drives me to always be my best, to always do unto others, to accept and embrace unconditionally. There are times in my life when I am undecided or afraid to go on. When I am able to let go of my fears, I find answers and total comfort. It is at these times I feel the endless love and support of my grandparents. I then have the opportunity to love, admire and respect them once again (in my memory, of course).

Gen's granddaughter, CA

~ I always felt that I'd let my Mom down because I was somewhat rebellious as a teenager. She was very controlling – her way of protecting me. But I didn't want to be protected; I wanted to get out and <u>do</u>. When caring for her during illness, I know I did the best I could and that makes me feel better about our relationship; that I made it up to her in some degree for all of the backtalk, worry, etc. I learned that I could organize just about anything. I found I have more patience than I needed to exhibit even with my two children. I have people who love me and care enough about me to listen to me go on and on about dealing with Mom and her issues many, many times. I believe in an afterlife because there just has to be something better for people who die after suffering an illness like AD.

Lanie's daughter, MN

YOUR THOUGHTS -

_____

_____

_____

_____

_____

_____

_____

_____

_____

_____

Extra journaling pages

Suggested reading:

1. **The Blue Day Book – A Lesson in Cheering Yourself Up**; Bradley Trevor Greive; 2000 – Andrews McMeel Publishing

2. **The 36 Hour Day - A Family Guide to Caring for Persons With Alzheimer Disease, Related Dementing Illnesses, and Memory Loss in Later Life**; Nancy L. Mace and Peter V. Rabins; 1999 – Johns Hopkins University Press/Warner Books

3. **Speaking Our Minds: Personal Reflections from Individuals With Alzheimer's;** Lisa Snyder; 2000 - Henry Holt & Company

4. **Partial View: An Alzheimer's Journal;** Cary Smith Henderson, Jackie Henderson Main, Ruth D. Henderson, Nancy Andrews; 1998 - Southern Methodist University Press

5. **Staying Connected While Letting Go: The Paradox of Alzheimer's Caregiving;** Sandy Braff, Mary Rose Olenick; 2003 - M. Evans and Company   (note: focuses on losing a spouse)

6. **Alive With Alzheimer's;** Cathy Stein Greenblat; 2004 - University of Chicago Press

7. **Consumer Reports Complete Guide to Health Services for Seniors: What Your Family Needs to Know About Finding and Financing, Medicare, Assisted Living, Nursing Homes, Home Care, Adult Day Care**; Trudy Lieberman, *Consumer Reports* Editors; 2000 – Three Rivers Press

8. **The Caregiver's Essential Handbook: More than 1,200 Tips to Help You Care for and Comfort the Seniors in Your Life;** Sasha Carr, Sandra Choron; 2003 - McGraw-Hill

9. **The House on Beartown Road: A Memoir of Learning and Forgetting**; Elizabeth Cohen; 2003 – Random House

10. **Alzheimer's: The Answers You Need**; Helen D. Davies, Helen Davies, Michael P. Jensen; 1998 – Elder Books

11. **Betty Crocker 4-Ingredient Dinners**; Betty Crocker (General Mills); 2003

12. Any book that offers encouragement.

13. Any book or movie that makes you laugh.

Resource List:

General Alzheimer's Information

1. **Alzheimer's Association**
   225 N. Michigan Ave., Fl. 17,
   Chicago, IL 60601
   24/7 Nationwide Contact Center: 1-800-272-3900
   www.alz.org

2. **Alzheimer's Disease Education and Referral Center (ADEAR)**
   (Affiliated with the National Institute on Aging – a U.S. government agency)
   ADEAR Center
   P.O. Box 8250
   Silver Springs, MD 20907-8250
   1-800-438-4380
   www.alzheimers.org

Caregiver Support

1. **National Association of Adult Day Services**
   (Affiliated with the National Council on Aging)
   409 3rd Street SW., Ste. 200
   Washington, DC 20024
   202-479-6682
   www.ncoa.org

2. **Caregiver Magazine (online articles – not necessary to subscribe)**
   www.caregiver.com

3. **General caregiving (some commercial aspects)**
   www.careguide.com

4. **National Family Caregivers Association**
   10400 Connecticut Ave., Ste. 500
   Kensington, MD 20895
   1-800-896-3650
   www.nfcacares.org

5. **AARP**
   601 E Street NW
   Washington, DC 20049
   www.aarp.org

Author's note: There are a number of websites that could be considered to be "helpful" for AD caregivers. However, there is a commercial aspect to them so I've not listed them here. If you'd like to find them, type "Alzheimer's caregivers" into a search engine and you'll get a good list to work with.

Important Phone Numbers and Addresses

Medical
Doctor: Name _____   Phone number _____

        Address _____   Nurse/Med. Assistant:

_____   _____

Dentist: Name _____   Phone number _____

        Address _____   Hygienist/Assistant:

_____   _____

Therapist: Name _____   Phone number _____

        Address _____   Assistant:

_____   _____

NOTES: _____

_____

Housing - Apartment

Manager: Name _____ Phone number _____

            Address _____ Secretary:

_____ _____

Maintenance: Name _____Phone number _____

            Address _____ Assistant:

_____ _____

Kitchen: Name _____ Phone number _____

            Address _____ Assistant:

_____ _____

Social
Worker: Name _____ Phone number _____

            Address _____ Manager:

_____ _____

Housing – Assisted Living

Manager: Name _____ Phone number _____

      Address _____ Secretary:

_____ _____

Nurse: Name _____ Phone number _____

      Address _____ Assistant:

_____ _____

Bookkeeping: Name _____ Phone number _____

      Address _____ Assistant:

_____ _____

Social
Worker: Name _____ Phone number _____

      Address _____ Manager:

_____ _____

Housing – Nursing Home

Nurses   Name _____ Phone number _____
Station:

      Address _____ Secretary:

_____ _____

Bookkeeping: Name _____ Phone number _____

      Address _____ Assistant:

_____ _____

Front desk: Name _____ Phone number _____

      Address _____ Assistant:

_____ _____

Social   Name _____ Phone number _____
Worker:

      Address _____ Manager:

_____ _____

Financial

Bank 1:   **Name** _____   **Phone number** _____

         Address _____   **Banker:**

_____   _____

Bank 2:   **Name** _____   **Phone number** _____

         Address _____   **Banker:**

_____   _____

Bank 3:   **Name** _____   **Phone number** _____

         Address _____   **Banker:**

_____   _____

Credit Union: **Name** _____   **Phone number** _____

         Address _____   **Assistant Manager:**

_____   _____

Transportation

Cab
Company

Name _____ Phone number _____

Address _____ Notes:

_____ _____

_____

Transit
Authority:

Name _____ Phone number _____

Address _____ Route/schedule:

_____ _____

_____

Garage:

Name_____ Phone number _____

Address _____ Mechanic:

_____ _____

_____

Airline:

Name _____ Phone number _____

Address _____ Notes:

_____ _____

_____

<u>Miscellaneous</u>

Beautician: Name_____ **Phone number** _____

    Address _____ **Stylist:**

_____   _____

Veterinarian: Name_____ **Phone number** _____

    Address _____ **Assistant:**

_____   _____

Newspaper: Name _____ **Phone number** _____

    Address _____ **Delivery schedule:**

_____   _____

Grocery   **Name**_____ **Phone number** _____
Delivery:

    Address _____ **Assistant Manager:**

_____   _____

Local   Name _____   Phone number _____
Alzheimer's
Assn. :   Address _____   Contact:

_____   _____

Counselor: Name _____   Phone number _____

Address _____   Contact:

_____   _____

Hospice: Name _____   Phone number _____

Address _____   Contact:

_____   _____

Hospital: Name _____   Phone number _____

Address _____   Room/Nursing Station:

_____   _____

Insurance Name_____ Phone number _____
Agency
      Address _____ Contact:

      _____ _____

Pension: Name _____ Phone number _____

      Address _____ Contact:

      _____ _____

Social   Name _____ Phone number _____
Security:
      Address _____ Contact:

      _____ _____

Medicare: Name _____ Phone number _____

      Address _____ Contact:

      _____ _____

Need Additional Copies of *Seasons of Good-bye: An Alzheimer's Caregiver Journal?*

Good news! You can order as many as you need directly from the publisher.

~ If paying by <u>check or money order</u>, <u>use this form.</u>
(Orders placed for shipping outside the U.S. must use the website below and pay by credit card.)

~ If paying with a <u>credit card</u> (VISA or MasterCard), log on to <u>www.alzjournal.com</u> for secure ordering with Verisign.

For purchase with check or money order (for your protection, **we do not accept cash**), kindly provide the following information (please print):

1. Name:_____

2. Mailing Address:_____

3. City_____ 4.State_____ 5. Zip_____

6. Daytime phone number (will be used only if there are questions about your order)   (   ) _____ -- _____

7. Number of books ordered: [   ]

8. Make check/money order payable to Halian Associates for **$9.95** ($10.60 for MN residents) per book. **ADD $2.25** for the first book ($1.50 for each additional book) to cover shipping and handling.

Mail this order form and your check/money order to: ⟹

Halian Associates
1292 Ferndale St. N.
Maplewood, MN 55119

Please allow 4 weeks for delivery.

VOLUME DISCOUNTS
For information regarding bulk order (more than ten books) discounts, please write to address at left or email alzbook@iglide.net

Holmes Associates
P.O. Box 28670
Oakdale, MN 55128